THE SECRET PRACTICE

EIGHTEEN YEARS ON THE DARK SIDE OF YOGA

JOELLE TAMRAZ

PARADISE PALM PUBLISHING

Copyright © 2023 by Joelle Tamraz - joelletamraz.com

Paradise Palm Publishing

ISBN-13: 978-1-7393777-0-0 (Paperback edition)

ISBN-13: 978-1-7393777-1-7 (Ebook edition)

British Library Cataloguing in Publication Data. A CIP record can be obtained for this book from the British Library.

First published 2023

Cover design: Kari Brownlie

Typesetting: Vellum

*For Mom, who never let me go
and for Trevor, who took my hand*

TABLE OF CONTENTS

PART IV
SEEDS OF LIFE

AUTHOR'S NOTE

Some names and identifying details have been changed to protect people's privacy. Otherwise, the story is true.

This book is appropriate for a general adult readership, however I'm mindful that certain passages may be triggering for someone who has experienced psychological abuse or coercive control.

PART I

YOGA MASTER

1

PRIVATE MARRIAGE

I pack my bags in a way that won't make him suspicious. Stuff everything inside: clothes, jewelry, books. I don't know how I'll carry it all, but whatever I don't take now, I'll lose forever. He hovers around me, watches my movements. I tell him I'm going to my mother's for a day. But I'm never coming back. I try to run, but my legs feel like they're moving through water. His hold, stronger than any he had in life, feels like a blanket pressed over my head. Suddenly I hear my own screams and the dogs barking. Drenched in sweat, my heart racing, I sit up, force in a breath, take in my surroundings.

I've already left.

TWENTY YEARS EARLIER, on the day of our marriage, I wanted Arun to stay forever. October sunlight danced in his eyes. He held my hands and asked for an exchange of promises ahead of our formal vows, one from each of us in honor of our special day. "I'll go first. Always tell me the truth."

That was easy. I was already true to him. "I will."

His navy-blue jacket hugged his torso. A scarf shielded his neck. He rubbed my hands. "Now you go."

I looked up into his deer eyes. "Never leave me."

No one knew we were getting married. No one except our landlord in the French town where I had come for my MBA. He and his wife had agreed to witness our union, and we sat, along with their two children, in the front row of a gold-corniced function room. Two grey-haired officials presided at a table covered in a white tablecloth, and if they wondered about our strange party, they didn't let on. They smiled and invited us to repeat our vows, then presented the documents we needed to sign to seal our bond. I stood next to Arun in my best outfit— an embroidered silk Indian suit he had bought for me in Delhi —my red hair half up in a single braid, my face flushed with joy. He pursed his lips and slid the gold band around my finger.

Our witnesses had surprised us with gifts: a glass decanter and a full-bellied, earth-toned vase. We went to drop them off at home before meeting at an Italian restaurant chosen that day. Their nine-year-old daughter came with us and sat next to me on the couch as Arun pulled up a chair in front of us. He peered at me through his glasses with an expression I knew well. "Congratulations on your marriage."

The girl giggled, and I turned to her and smiled.

Tao had arrived. I could see the glow in Arun's face, his jagged edges disappear as Tao spoke: "We were all there. Even Baba. If you had been more aware, you would have felt us."

The elders who governed Arun's life. He had never channeled anyone other than Tao but referred to the eight of them often. Tao was suggesting I had missed something exceptional; the whole pantheon of Arun's hidden world was a rare, perhaps unique, occurrence, but I had been too focused on the most important day of my life to sense their presence. I had been immersed in the moment. My moment.

"We all want to wish you well."

I smiled and bowed my head slightly with respect. The girl looked down, quiet.

Soon after, we left the apartment and joined her family for pasta and pizza on red-checked tablecloths.

When Arun and I returned home later in the afternoon, the last rays of sunshine filtered through the skylights. The apartment was quiet. Sitting alone at the dining table on one side of the living room, I contemplated the day. It had been perfect. Simple, spontaneous, entirely ours. Just as I had wanted. It didn't matter that my parents weren't there. It was better this way. I had never dreamed of walking down the aisle hooked on Dad's arm, wearing a long white gown, a church full of people looking on. What I had sought I had received: the true love of an enlightened man.

For months, we guarded our union from the forces that would seek to destroy it and kept our marriage secret from my friends and family. When the news dropped in a phone conversation with Mom, I braced myself for her fury. The line was quiet for a moment, then her voice sounded calm.

"You didn't think it was a good idea to tell me?"

"I didn't think you'd want to know."

"I wish I had seen you on your wedding day."

Her melancholy tone surprised me. Why did she want to be there? She hated Arun. The man who was the same age as Dad, thirty-three years older than me.

2

THE ROAD TO RISHIKESH

W hen I met Arun at the age of twenty-two, I had already been practicing New Age and Eastern meditation for over ten years. It started with Actualism. Mom took my sister Saby and me to learn at a musty center in a hotel on the west side of New York City. The three of us were connected like the angles of a triangle, and she wanted to include us in her own explorations. Saby, who was only three and too young to learn, spent her time coloring while I took private lessons with a sweet blond-haired woman. I liked her and listened intently as she described the crown of colored lights on my head and how to invoke the appropriate light based on its property. The session ended with a long, tape-recorded lecture by the founder of Actualism. He spoke in a calm monotone, and I tried hard not to nod off.

By my mid-teens, my teacher announced that she was moving out of state. I was disappointed to see her go and resolved to ask her a question that had been on my mind for some time. "Are the colors real?"

Her usually impassive face creased into a frown. "Of course

they're real. What do you think I've been teaching you all these years?"

I looked down. I hadn't meant to offend her, but how could she expect me to believe in a literal crown of colored lights?

I invoked the colors from time to time over my high school years, especially the blue one for mental clarity before exams, but had no further spiritual instruction until I turned eighteen, and Mom took us to learn Transcendental Meditation, commonly known as TM. She had seen its positive effects on a friend and wanted us to share the experience with her. Saby was nine and joined the children's group while Mom and I shuffled into a crowded room of adults. Our instructors, who looked like conventional middle-aged Americans, described the field of universal consciousness, from which all goodness was meant to emanate, with the certitude of a science. They played videos of Maharishi Mahesh Yogi, meaning "great seer greatest yogi": a diminutive Indian man, dressed in a white robe, with long greying locks and a beard. He spoke in a methodical high-pitched voice punctuated by the occasional giggle and shared the wonders we would soon discover. Creative intelligence, a deep sense of calm, inner joy, and radiant health were all within our reach. He had left the tranquility of his Himalayan home to offer his unique gift to the world, and we were the lucky ones to receive it. The course fee of several hundred dollars couldn't compare to what we would learn.

The practice itself was deceptively simple. We were given a secret personal mantra that we had to repeat silently for twenty minutes twice a day while sitting with a straight back, eyes closed. When our thoughts wandered from our mantra, we should be gentle with ourselves and simply return to the repetition.

On the evening of our instruction, while Mom and I sat

together in the kitchen, she looked at me with a mischievous smile. "What's your mantra?"

"Mom, we're not supposed to tell anyone."

"I'll tell you mine." She leaned in and whispered two syllables sounding vaguely Chinese.

I waited a moment, then did the same.

I felt no different for having told her; there were no apparent consequences for violating the code of secrecy.

I kept the method in the back of my mind throughout the summer but rarely practiced. It was the last time I could enjoy the city with my friends before starting university at Harvard. I would never be as free from cares or worries again. But when September came around and Mom dropped me off at my campus dorm, I felt unmoored and decided to commit to a regular practice of TM to keep me grounded. I rarely managed an afternoon meditation but never skipped the twenty minutes to start the day.

Unlike some of the other students, there wasn't an obvious group I could join. I was born in Lebanon of Lebanese-Egyptian parents who had immigrated to France when I was two. They hadn't taught me Arabic. Our family was Catholic, but after I left Paris for New York at the age of nine, my Sunday church attendance, once instilled by my French governess, Maselle, was reduced to twice-a-year family visits at Easter and Christmas. By the time I reached Harvard, my concept of God was conjoined with the light of Actualism and the universal consciousness of TM.

I looked up the local TM center in Cambridge and soon started attending the weekly group meditation, followed by a copious homemade vegetarian dinner. A friendly welcoming couple, as conventional as the instructors in New York, ran the place. I enjoyed the warm space and felt comfortable socializing with people of all ages around a shared practice.

One evening, as I walked back to my dorm after a group

meditation and dinner, I contemplated the dome of darkness and faraway stars above me and felt a deep connection to the universe and my place in it. As a child I had sometimes felt acutely alone, watching my parents and their extravagant lifestyle from a distance, and though I didn't know what my destiny would be, meditation had connected me to the spiritual purpose of my life.

I met James the first time I went to the TM center. He wasn't part of the regular group but emerged from the basement reserved for advanced practitioners. With his shoulder-length black curls and wiry beard, he looked like a younger version of Maharishi and stood out from all the other meditators. A visiting mathematics professor fifteen years my senior, he spoke in slow breathy tones. I didn't feel an immediate physical attraction toward him but was fascinated by the depth of his spiritual knowledge. His longing to uncover hidden truths resonated with mine.

Within weeks, we were dating.

When I brought him home to meet my family, Mom was taken by him in a similar way. He sat at the edge of her bed to speak with her, and she leaned against her pillows and confided in him.

"Since the girls' father left, I haven't found the right man to share my life."

She rarely spoke with me in such an intimate way, and I tried not to focus on them.

After he had visited several times, she told me she had asked him if he had used spiritual power to attract me.

"He said he did."

I was shocked by the admission, but she didn't offer any more clues, and I didn't know if she was worried or impressed.

James encouraged both Mom and me to take the advanced meditation course known as the TM-Siddhis. It cost three thousand dollars, but he said he wouldn't recommend such an expense if it wasn't worth it. *Siddhis* means perfections in Sanskrit but is also interpreted as yogic powers in the *Yoga Sutras of Patanjali*, a foundational text. The advanced TM course promised to teach us how to harness these powers, including the most famous: yogic flying. The practice appeared to be a propulsive hop from the meditation mattress. It was shrouded in mystery, but the promise that we might learn how to perform this feat was tantalizing. Mom signed up that summer.

She returned with the full weight of her experience. She had been one of the first to fly and spoke to James in hushed tones. He listened with his eyes glued on her. They were now members of an exclusive elite society, and I left them to their private exchange.

Eager to join their ranks, I signed up the following summer, after my second year at Harvard. I didn't feel I could ask Mom for the money on top of the tuition and living expenses she was already paying, so I turned to Dad. He and Mom had separated when I was nine, shortly after Saby's birth, and divorced seven years later. He had been an unreliable presence throughout my life, showing up unannounced and disappearing in the same way, but since his divorce from Mom, our relationship was even more distant. He traveled around the world chasing deals, and the least he could do was help me once in a while. I called to tell him about the course and ask him for money.

He responded, "I don't believe in such things."

"I really want to do it."

"If it's so important to you." He was reluctant but at least he had agreed.

The two-week residential course was held at a hotel, with women separate from men at all times. In a large conference room covered in mattresses, surrounded by my cohort of female meditators, I learned to repeat the *siddhis*, Sanskrit phrases translated into English, over and over in my mind. We could sit in whatever position we wanted and I chose to kneel, but couldn't imagine how repeating the phrase "lightness of cotton," would magically propel me into the air.

Over the course of the first week, then into the second, one woman after another took a first hop, whether cross-legged or kneeling. My mind merged into the group's focus, and eventually I felt the same propulsion. My hops filled me with a sense of relief: I had reached Mom's level—not one of the first, but it didn't matter now.

By my third year at Harvard, James's hold on me weakened. He had returned to his job in Europe six months earlier and became increasingly focused on esoteric spiritual pursuits beyond TM. He read *Autobiography of a Yogi*—one of the first books about yoga written for a western audience and published in 1946—and became entranced with the figure of Babaji, described as a master yogi who had overcome death, lived for centuries in a youthful body, and now dwelled in a state of permanent transcendence. James bought me a copy of the book, and though I didn't share his interest in the obscure arts of levitation, mental projection, and eternal life, I looked up to the long dark-haired androgynous youth. We attended a different kind of meditation workshop, and I returned with a line drawing of Babaji, which I placed on the bookshelf above my desk. Along with the Maharishi of TM, whose image crowned the altar I had created in my room from stacked boxes and a sheet, Babaji presided over my daily life.

My veneration for yoga masters notwithstanding, I had no plans to ever visit their native country, but through my major in social studies and my interest in religion and economic development, I met an academic advisor specializing in South Asian cultures. Under his guidance, I wrote my senior thesis on Gandhi-inspired social activism in India and traveled there for field research. James, hoping to rekindle our relationship, joined me and suggested a stop in Rishikesh at the end of the trip. I had never heard of the place, but he knew it as the ancient abode of the yogis, a town made famous in the sixties by The Beatles' visit to their then-guru, the Maharishi of TM.

In the lowest foothills of the Himalayas across the two banks of the roaring grey-green Ganges, Rishikesh is an impressive mountain location. When we visited in the early nineties, both Indian and foreign tourists flocked to its spiritual establishments, known as ashrams. Only a few abandoned huts remained of the Maharishi's ashram, but we found a room at the prominent Sivananda ashram, one of the few that welcomed foreign visitors.

Toward the end of our stay, we met a man, the brother of one of Mom's friends, who had left the TM movement after reaching its senior ranks and joined the Sivananda ashram. Years of yogic hopping had left his knees injured, and he was disillusioned not only with the TM-Siddhis but also with the whole global organization for promoting such harmful teachings. He cited the warning in Patanjali's *Yoga Sutras* that attachment to yogic powers is a hindrance to the path of enlightenment. His argument made sense to me: the propulsion to fly now seemed like a misguided human endeavor, not a meaningful spiritual goal. Soon after we met, I abandoned the TM-Siddhis meditation and never returned to it.

When I left Rishikesh that summer, my feelings for James remained lukewarm. I hadn't enjoyed the austere life at the Sivananda ashram and didn't imagine I would return.

At the end of my fourth and final year of university, I applied for a travel grant on a whim. My thesis on Gandhian activism had received muted responses, and though I gave up my goal of becoming a professor of anthropology, I was still intrigued by Indian spirituality. I applied for jobs in the business sector, and as I had heard nothing more about the grant, accepted an offer in business consulting at a local firm. A few days later, the awarding committee got in touch to say that the winner had declined the grant, and it was mine should I want it. Fate had dealt me an extraordinary hand. When would someone ever offer me money to travel again? The next morning, I accepted the grant and contacted the consulting company to delay my start date by six months.

By my graduation, it was clear to James that my attraction to him had waned irreversibly, but we remained friends, and I asked him to travel with me to India a second time. I wanted a companion to help me navigate the highly sexist culture, at least for the start of the journey, and didn't know anyone else who would want to go. Despite initial resistance, when I offered to pay for his plane ticket, he agreed. After all, there was much he still wanted to learn from India.

On our first night in Delhi, I lay on the hotel sheets past midnight as the overhead fan whirled at low speed and the smell of mothballs filled the air. I was in India again—on the other side of the world—against all odds. The wonder and excitement of my surroundings kept me awake until the sounds of revving vehicles dwindled, and a few hours later I awoke to the honk of scooters and rays of sunshine piercing through the flimsy curtains.

After a few days in Delhi, we returned to Rishikesh. I hadn't found what I wanted in the capital and knew exactly where we would stay this time: the Ganges Guest House, a clean and simple accommodation managed by a Swiss woman married to an Indian swami (the general term used to denote a Hindu male belonging to a religious order). Their accommodation was much more inviting than the grey halls of Sivananda ashram.

On this second visit, Rishikesh felt much more familiar. Our day was structured around a walk along the unpaved path by the river, green hills rising all around us. As we crossed the long suspension bridge, swamis in their saffron robes clanged coins in their brass bowls. The further bank was filled with ashrams, shops, and restaurants, the smell of incense mingling with frying oil. I lingered in bookstores redolent of printing ink and perused floor-to-ceiling shelves while enjoying a break from the moist heat in the cool air of ceiling fans.

After the endless bustle of Delhi, I merged into the serene pace of life and had no plans for further travel, but James was bent upon encountering Babaji, who he thought lived in a cave near Badrinath, the major Hindu pilgrimage site in the north. It seemed unlikely to me that the supreme yoga master would make an appearance for us. Locals warned us not to travel into the high Himalayas in September, as there was still a risk of landslides at the tail end of the monsoon, but with only a couple of weeks before his return to his job in Europe, James was adamant.

Within hours of setting off, the bus stopped in the middle of the mountains as the road ahead was blocked by a landslide, and all the passengers disembarked in an unknown village at dusk. James and I were the only foreigners. There was no guest house in the village, and we had nowhere to go, so we sat at the bus stand to catch our bearings. Before we had time to worry about what to do next, the local police chief came to our side and took us to his home. He opened an unused garden room and cheerfully offered to let us stay there until the road cleared. Though the room was filled with thick layers of dust, it was separate from the rest of the house and had a bed. The water pipes leading into the village had been crushed, and there was no running water for the duration of our stay. I can't imagine what would have happened to us if he hadn't extended his welcome.

Three days later we got word that the bus could move and resumed the journey to Badrinath. At an elevation of over 3,000 meters, the mountains were covered only in shrubs, and gusts of cold wind swept through the valley; my thin clothes and the synthetic shawl I had bought along the way were no match for the elements. Our quest seemed even less promising than when we had set off, but James was undeterred. As soon as we had dropped our bags at a guest house, we left for his mission to find Babaji.

To reach the mountains, we had to pass by the temple that was the main attraction for pilgrims. Throngs pressed between carts filled with brass figurines of gods and cones of the bright red tilak powder used to mark the forehead. James didn't waste a minute and asked someone for Babaji's whereabouts. The local pointed in the general direction of the mountain range, but I doubted he knew anything about the mythical yoga master James had in mind. How I wished I could stay in the safety of people rather than follow him into the unknown barren terrain. We left the pilgrims and ventured into desolate crags. The only sound was James's voice calling out "Babaji" into the whistling wind. As the light started to dim, fatigue and worry overcame me. We had hiked for over an hour with absolutely nothing around us. I called an end to the search, and we returned to the guest house.

That night I fell into a heavy mindless sleep and awoke the next morning with a tightness in my chest and a congested cough. After washing up and getting dressed, I said to James, "I need to leave."

He looked at me in disbelief. "We only just arrived."

"I know, but I'm sick, and I won't be able to recover if I stay here. I'm too cold."

He looked as if I had betrayed him; but I ignored him, walked to the bus stand, and inquired about the timing of the next bus to Rishikesh. When I returned to our room to pick up my bag, James didn't say a word, but he followed me to the bus stop, a few steps behind.

As the bus hurtled down the mountain range, swerving through hairpin bends, I felt buoyant despite the heaviness in my head and chest. Soon, we would be back in the warmth and comfort of Rishikesh. I would have left without James if he had insisted on staying. His search was futile—we wouldn't find Babaji in those mountains—and I was done with his risky undertaking. Back at the guest house, I bought a gas cylinder for my room and made several cups of tea a day. After visiting a local doctor who diagnosed me with a common cold, I started to feel better, eased into a peaceful routine, and recovered slowly.

One afternoon, several days after our return, I went to retrieve a towel I had left to dry on the balcony, but it wasn't there. I walked down the stairs to the foyer and saw a man sitting in the shadows of dusk. His hands clasped in his lap, his gaze set in the middle distance, his toes curled gracefully under a white plastic armchair. His t-shirt and thin shorts, though of the salmon-orange color of the swamis, didn't match the attire of a holy man. I tried to place him, but his thin aquiline nose, shoulder-length greying curls, and bronze skin suggested a range of countries from the Mediterranean to India. He sat absorbed in a state of calm, and I assumed he hadn't seen me, but then he turned suddenly. "What can I do for you?"

His attention and direct question caught me off-guard. "Nothing. My towel fell from the balcony."

Without pause he addressed the hotel attendant, who came into my field of vision then. "Son, go fetch this lady's towel."

He spoke in Hindi, but I could understand what he said. He was poised, dignified, in complete command. I fell under his spell.

3

AN AMERICAN YOGI

James and I met him again the following evening. The sun had set—the Ganges invisible outside the windows —and a faint smell of incense lingered in the air. We joined him, along with a coterie of female tourists, sitting around a white plastic table. He introduced himself as Swami Arun and asked about us. I told him about my research on Gandhian notions of truth and nonviolence and my desire to explore their religious underpinnings.

He responded in a brash tone. "Gandhi was bad for India. Because of his negotiations with the British, the nation was divided, and millions of people died."

I had never heard anyone voice this opinion and sat up in my seat. His accent was unusual, but it was clear he was Indian, and I didn't want to argue about his country.

He dominated the group conversation, and when we returned to our room, James said, "That man knows something. I like his smile."

The next day, he went to meet him privately, and as he was leaving, I said, "Ask him if he has a girlfriend."

He returned an hour later, delighted by his exchange and

despondent about returning to Europe just when he had finally met a genuine spiritual master. And no, he didn't have a girl-friend: he had had many women in his life, but he was single now.

The following morning at dawn, I walked to the shared bathroom down the hall wearing a t-shirt and a towel around my waist, not expecting to see anyone. Swami Arun emerged from the opposite direction, his hair loose and eyes unfocused. As we crossed paths, his gaze met mine for a moment, and I felt exposed in my attire. I would take greater care in the future, no matter the time of day; rules of female propriety were strict in India.

JAMES LEFT SOON AFTER, a month into my four-month stay in India. I watched his taxi pull away from the rubble in front of the guest house. When the car had disappeared in the distance, I dragged myself back to the empty room we had shared, sat at the table, and cupped my warm hands over my eyes. It was an exercise I had learned with him, and as my mind rested in the dark, I imagined him arriving in Delhi, boarding his flight, then returning to the world we knew.

In our final days together, he had wanted to practice semen retention with me. He had read in the yogic lore how holding off ejaculation during intercourse confers exceptional energy, health, and spiritual bliss. His efforts on the flimsy mattress of my single bed felt perverse, his goal as unreachable as his search for Babaji. In his progression toward increasingly esoteric practices, semen retention was the low point. I put an end to all sexual contact.

I had been ready for him to leave but still felt unprepared for the unmooring—the inner hollowness—of those first moments alone. I would need to find my own path in a culture whose workings I barely grasped. To calm my anxiety, I made a mental inventory of all the people I knew in Rishikesh: the white-bearded Spanish man who kept striking up conversations but didn't inspire my confidence; Julia, the other foreign woman, who would be joining me on a course at the Sivananda Ashram Forest Academy. We had both been in the audience when the senior swami announced a formal yoga course open exclusively to Indian men. I had inched forward on my knees, bowed my head before him, and asked to be included as an exception. With his beak-like nose and head covered in a scarf, he had stared ahead for a moment, then granted my request. When Julia followed with her own, he accepted her as well. The only two women in a class of men, we would surely become friends.

Just as my thoughts started to settle, someone knocked on the door. I wasn't expecting anyone but had no reason to worry and went to open. There with his large hand pressed into the jamb was Swami Arun.

He grinned and spoke with a drawl. "Are you alright?"

I smiled at his unexpected friendly presence. "Yes, I'm fine."

"I just wanted to check on you."

I was touched by his concern and surprised that he had thought about me.

He invited me to lunch at a well-known local restaurant along with the group of female tourists. I thanked him but declined, as I had already ordered my meal at the guest house.

He shook his head. "I can't eat the food here. It always arrives cold."

I nodded with understanding but preferred the simplicity of a home-cooked meal to the richness of restaurant food. As I shut the door, I couldn't help but cheer up.

Swami Arun, how could I have forgotten him?

. . .

HE RETURNED every day that week and renewed his lunch invitation with a warm glowing smile. I declined each time for the same reason but made sure to show appreciation. One evening he knocked on my door with a different message. "Your mother's on the line." His voice was caring and familiar, as if he knew both Mom and me.

I ran down the stairs to the reception desk and picked up the only phone at the guest house. Mom's upbeat voice flowed over the line, and we spoke for close to an hour. When she expressed concern, I repeated, "Everything is fine, Mom." My mood lifted, and I didn't mind that everyone in the foyer, including Swami Arun and the other tourists, could overhear my conversation.

The next day I decided to skip the guest house meal and offered to join him for lunch. We walked to the restaurant across the river and took a table for two. When his usual group of female companions arrived a few minutes later, he glanced in their direction but didn't ask them to join us. I felt special, flattered by his singular interest in me, and wanted to know more about this man with the triumphant smile.

I spoke about the yoga course, which I would be joining soon, and the special dispensation I had received from the senior swami.

"You mean that sick man?"

I didn't understand.

"You know he has leprosy, right?"

The old swami always had his head wrapped in a scarf, and the skin underneath looked discolored, but I didn't expect him to have such a serious disease.

Swami Arun clasped his hands and rubbed one thumb over the other, his fingers thick and long like small sausages, apart from his thumbs with their half-moon nails filling the whole of the top joint. He seemed pleased with the knowledge he had dropped without warning.

I met him in the evenings with the other tourists, but our talks remained social. He told us with a grin how locals didn't believe he was Indian. "They think I'm American. I have to show them my passport."

These snippets of conversation left me wanting more; I longed to learn about the spiritual knowledge he guarded. One evening, I decided to overcome my natural shyness and went to find him after buying my usual drink of warm milk. He had moved into a larger room with a private bathroom on the top floor, and when I knocked on his door he opened as if he had been expecting me. His space was brightly lit and fully inhabited. On the table he had a red apple with a bite taken out of it, a bowl of fresh cream, and a bar of Cadbury milk chocolate (the only brand available in India, it felt like an exclusive treat). A popular adventure novel lay open face down on the bedside table. The array of familiar yet enticing objects, along with his welcoming smile, put me at ease.

He invited me to sit on the chair and perched himself on the edge of his bed, then cast a suspicious glance at my glass of milk. "I can't drink milk. But if I tell you why, you won't be able to drink it either."

I smiled with closed lips. There was nothing he could tell me that would change my mind about milk.

He told me I could dispense with his title and call him Arun, then spoke about his life since leaving India in the sixties. He had started in Saudi Arabia, where he welded oil pipelines, then moved to Germany, where he found work delivering newspapers. He arrived in New York a few years later, worked in construction—lofts downtown—and lived in hotels for singles. He liked the city and had no plans to move until a friend suggested a trip to Los Angeles. By his second visit, he stayed there for good.

In LA, his life really came together. He gave massages based on what he had learned from his Himalayan masters and built a lucrative business. He spoke with relish about how he worked from the early hours to mid-morning, then had the day to himself. He read the newspaper over coffee and took long bike rides on the beach.

He had moved back to India a year earlier and already made a name for himself in Rishikesh by working on Swami Chidananda, one of the illustrious leaders of Sivananda ashram, whom he described as a noble man of great learning, born without sexual desire.

"I healed his shoulder pain, and he didn't want to be without me. I stayed with him two weeks, then I left. I'm nobody's servant." His eyes opened wide, and I listened to his stories as if I were resuming a conversation with an old friend. He didn't say what had brought him back to India after decades abroad, but I gathered it was a momentous shift after a long spell of good fortune. Maybe we were both travelers who had found each other at the right time.

He asked about me, and I told him about my Middle Eastern roots, then growing up in New York after Saby was born.

"I think I saw you there. In the eighties."

He paused to let me take in the information. I doubted that it was possible or that he would recognize me from childhood.

"I just came down from my cave in Gangotri. I was in meditation and fasted for forty days. Then the elders told me I had to come here. I didn't want to, but they insisted."

His fast explained the muscle-to-bone leanness of his strong frame. I sensed his veneration for the elders, his guides in this life, and beyond.

"I teach an authentic yoga from the Himalayas. Only to specific students. Not in groups. I might be able to teach you."

These were the words I had been wanting to hear. I sensed his intimate connection to the divine, and as if reading my thoughts, he said, "What if I showed you God in the next room? What would you do then?"

The idea of seeing God in a literal way frightened me, like Moses with the burning bush. I wasn't ready for that kind of direct vision.

"People say, 'God, God.' But what do they do? How do they change?"

True: knowing God didn't mean anything unless a person changed their behavior accordingly.

"You should read the Quran."

"I'm not Muslim."

"What religion are you?"

"Christian."

"You should read the Bible then. Everyone should know their own holy book."

I nodded.

"Come to me tomorrow morning at five."

I wanted to know everything there was to know about him, and I was ready to learn whatever he would teach me.

I had been there a while, and his eyes were bloodshot. I glanced at the clock on the bedside table: close to eleven. We had spoken for three hours, and I hadn't felt the time pass. But it was way past our bedtime and time for me to go.

He fixed his gaze on me a final time. "You will have three sons, and I will hold your firstborn son in my arms."

In the palpable stillness of the night, I let his prophecy settle in my mind. Three sons sounded like a blessing for a certain kind of woman. But not for me. A different calling tugged at my soul. I felt God's presence. I was in India again, and I had met an authentic yogi. The answer came to me in the silence of my mind.

There are no sons in my future, but I will know you for the rest of my life.

4

YOGA LESSONS AT DAWN

My alarm woke me earlier than usual, and I pulled myself out of bed, opened the balcony door, and inhaled the smell of burning wood. After washing up, I put on my cutoff flannel shorts, loose t-shirt, and worn flip-flops, and walked up to Arun's room. After only a few hours of sleep, I knocked on his door at five.

He looked bewildered to see me, as if he had forgotten his invitation from the night before. I stood still, undeterred, until he let me in and asked me to sit. The air in his room carried a hint of smoke—incense perhaps. He went into the bathroom at the back, and when he reappeared, the haze had lifted from his face. He pulled up another seat and turned to me. "Do you know the myth of the churning of the ocean?"

I had studied it at Harvard in a Hindu mythology class. "Yes."

"Tell it to me."

In the instant, I didn't know where to start. "I can't remember the details."

The room was dim, and his voice was low and measured with a nasal tone.

"When the gods and the demons wanted to extract the nectar of immortality buried in the ocean, they placed Mount Meru on a tortoise, who was Lord Vishnu. Then they wrapped a snake around the mountain and tugged from each side. The demons held the fiery mouth, and the gods took the tail. First a poison came up. The lord Shiva swallowed it, and it turned his throat blue. That's why he's sometimes called *nilkanth*. After some time, they reached the nectar."

I sat rapt and listened.

"This is just a myth, but it explains in images the process I will teach you. The mountain is the spine. The tortoise is the pelvis. The snake represents kundalini, the energy at the base of the spine. Churning the ocean is the process of breathing. The gods and the demons are inside us; right and left, our divine and human tendencies."

At his decoding of the ancient myth, my desire to learn bloomed.

"My masters were Chinese. They lived at the border between China and India. Everything I know comes from them. The Indian yogis focused on the immortality of the soul, but the Chinese took it further. They developed the process of physical longevity."

The first grey light of dawn filtered through the window. He gazed at me.

"You will need to be patient. When the poison comes up, you will hate me. But if you stick with the practice, you will reach the nectar. Don't stop, no matter how much you hate me."

He sounded serious, concerned even, but I couldn't imagine hating him.

He got up. "Sit on the floor. Any way you are comfortable."

I kneeled.

He came down next to me.

"The most powerful breathing in the world is slow, even breathing through the nose. Inhale so slowly you don't feel

25

the air passing through your nostrils. Exhale in the same way."

I closed my eyes and focused on the movement of air, concentrating until its passage became almost imperceptible, Arun's gentle presence beside me.

After a couple of minutes, he stopped me. "How did you feel?"

"Good. Calm."

"That's enough for today. Come back tomorrow."

I couldn't believe my good fortune; I had traveled so far to learn precisely this.

The next morning, he said he needed to balance my solar plexus before any further teaching. "It's a requirement for yoga to work, but these modern teachers don't even know about it. The original knowledge was lost."

He asked me to lie on his bed and pulled up my t-shirt with a quick tug, like a doctor conducting a medical examination, then gathered his fingers and pressed them into my navel. Although I trusted him, I didn't like having my belly exposed. I tried to relax, but as his fingers dug deeper, I yelped.

"Sorry." He released the pressure a bit but left his fingers in place. "Very out of balance."

"What's wrong?"

"There should be a clear heartbeat directly under the navel. Yours is out of place."

He massaged my belly in concentric circles and explained that an off-center heartbeat could lead to all kinds of physical disturbances, from constipation to physical weakness and emotional distress. Then he stopped and felt for the pulse again. Still dissatisfied, he asked me to raise my joined legs at a forty-five-degree angle. My belly ballooned out, and my back arched. When it felt like I couldn't hold my legs in place any longer, he finally told me to bring them down and said I would need one more adjustment.

I wanted to be healed.

"You can't experience the benefits of yoga if the energy is not flowing properly in the body. These priests and swamis who pray in the morning while constipated don't know anything."

We moved to the floor, and he explained the heart of his teaching.

"The most important part of the process is reverse abdominal breathing. Breathe in, stomach in. Breathe out, stomach out. The opposite of how we breathe all the time."

He inhaled and pulled his abdominal muscles in and up, hollowing out his belly, held his breath for a moment, then exhaled and pushed his abdominal muscles down so his lower belly expanded. "Now you try."

I practiced a few breaths under his observation.

"Keep it up all the time. Whenever you remember. Not just once a day in the morning."

I nodded.

"Now I'll show you physical exercises."

I told him I only wanted to learn the spiritual aspect of yoga. I had taken two different yoga classes at a gym in New York, and neither one had convinced me to keep up the practice. The first was a series of separate poses I could perform with ease, and the other was athletic and repetitive; neither one led to the absorption I felt during meditation.

"We can't separate the physical part from the spiritual. If the body is in pain, you can't meditate. Healthy mind in a healthy body."

He showed me a long bamboo pole, placed it on his shoulders, and extended his arms on either end. With his wrists wrapped over the pole and his feet aligned, he bent from side to side.

Then he handed me the pole. "Now you try."

I placed it at the base of my neck and stretched my arms

over it as he had done. He watched my movements and corrected the alignment of my shoulder and arms. The side bends exerted a gentle stretch on my lower back.

He took the pole again, placed it on his shoulders, and this time twisted in the horizontal plane. When it was my turn, he instructed me to keep my feet planted on the floor and my head facing forward to limit the twisting movement.

After a while, he asked, "How do you feel?"

"I like the exercises." The assisted deep stretching had been pleasant.

"I just invented this series. It's different from other movements. It opens the space between the vertebrae. I'll get a stick cut for you in your size."

It was easy to follow his plan, his steady focus and confidence.

As my lessons continued each morning, he layered on the energetic aspect of the process. He taught me to sit cross-legged on the floor, with my left heel tucked under my pelvis and my right foot in front of it. The meditation pose is known as *siddhasana*, the pose of perfection.

"Your heel should press into the perineum, the small muscle between the anus and the vagina. As you inhale, contract the perineum. This is the root lock, known as *mula bandha*. As you exhale, release the lock."

It took me a while to feel comfortable balancing on my left heel; but once I got used to it, it felt stable.

"Now drop your head and stretch your neck so your chin comes to your chest. This is the throat lock. Inhale and contract the perineum. Pull the energy up the spine. Exhale, release the lock, and move the energy down the front."

I practiced a few times; head bent, eyes closed.

"You can stop now."

I raised my head, buzzing with energy from the controlled breathing and muscle contractions.

"How do you feel?"

"Focused. Concentrated."

"Keep practicing like this as much as you like. Just make sure you move the energy up the back and then down the front. If you go up the front, it will increase sexual desire."

He sounded serious. I considered his words in silence. Sexuality and enlightenment—the twin poles of human desire. Yoga seemed to flirt with both, but I knew why I was there: liberation from the cycle of pain; enlightenment as defined by the Buddha, which I had studied in a seventh-grade history class on world religions.

"How long do I need to practice?"

"There's no hard and fast rule. Do it as long as you like. In time, a ball will drop from your perineum. You will feel it there. It's proof of the progress."

I practiced every day on my own, after my TM mantra meditation, but soon I dropped the TM part. It felt shallow compared to the subtle physical sensations and heightened awareness of the controlled breathing process synchronized with the root and throat locks. My body became a tight vessel of energy and vibrations, breathing like the flow of the tides, continuous and hypnotic.

"I can never teach this yoga to a group," he said during a lesson. "Each student has different abilities. I'm glad I found someone I can teach."

I thought about James, how much he had wanted to learn from Arun. Too bad he had missed the opportunity.

Into my second week of learning, Arun hadn't mentioned payment for his teaching, so I assumed it was free, his sole reward a worthy student. Then one morning at the end of my lesson, he spoke of serving his masters for twelve years—the price he had paid for the knowledge. "We don't have that kind of time in the modern world. I will teach you for three thousand dollars."

The sudden mention of a staggering amount, the same fee as the TM-Siddhis course, was totally unexpected after his praise of my ability, and he must have detected my sense of shock. "My normal fee is six thousand, but you're learning very well. I would teach you for free, but you wouldn't value the teaching. People only value what they pay for."

His expression was gentle and knowing, and my earlier assumption about learning for free now seemed presumptuous.

"There's no pressure. If you don't want to continue, you won't owe me anything for what I taught you so far."

I hadn't spoken with James since his return to Europe, but that afternoon I called and told him I was learning from Arun and he had requested a large payment.

"Are you sure of his intentions toward you?"

I frowned at the insinuation. "Yes, I'm completely sure."

I ended the conversation quickly and returned to my room. Sex again. Why would Arun ask for payment if he wanted to have sex with me?

He was nothing like Chandra-swami, the corrupt guru James and I had met in our first days in Delhi. With his white robe and red dot on his forehead, he had caught my attention in the elevator of my mother's building in New York. He had gleaming dark hair and stern eyes but responded to my namaste gesture with an invitation to visit him at the penthouse apartment where he was staying. I knew his host from my parents and took him up on the offer. I was shown to his room, and after we chatted for a while, he invited me to his ashram in Delhi. Before I left, he played a game of mind reading—correctly guessing when I thought about a rose, then the number seven—but it left me unimpressed. I wanted to plumb the secrets of the universe, not be the subject of a magic trick.

In Delhi, we learned the truth about this white-robed

swami. On the day we arrived at this ashram, an opulent mansion manned by armed guards, I was summoned alone to his room, and he offered to teach me his secret yoga, which included tantric sex with men of his choice. Shocked by his proposal, and my own gullibility, I didn't sleep that night, though I had insisted on sharing a room with James. We left in a hurry the following morning, and I didn't relax until we reached Rishikesh. Even then, I had nightmares for several nights that Chandra-swami had hunted me down.

Arun was nothing like Chandra-swami. He was a man my father's age who had lived in the US for years and taken on my instruction with calm focus and attention. Someday I would tell him about my dangerous mistake in Delhi.

Back in my room, I fished out the envelope Dad had given me from the bottom of my backpack. I had visited him and his wife Lena in Paris before traveling to India, and he had come to find me on my last day. "I wish I could have gone to India with you. I'll come to see you in Delhi on my way to China." He was driven by his relentless travels and hectic schedule of important meetings, and it hadn't crossed my mind that he would consider traveling with me, a trip of no financial value to him. Had he told me earlier, I wouldn't have asked James.

He handed me a thick envelope. "Here, take this. In case you need it."

I thanked him for his gift—thirty crisp hundred-dollar bills. I didn't think I would need it. I already had traveler's checks to cover my expenses in India. But now something unexpected had happened. The next morning, I gave the envelope to Arun.

5

BABA'S HEIR

As the monsoon humidity lifted and the autumn sunshine emerged, the world I uncovered with Arun in the plain decor of his guest house room was filled with men achieving exceptional personal feats.

"Originally, yoga was created for men so they could please women and make love for a long time," he explained.

I knew about James's semen-retention experiments, and indeed there was no mention of women in the original texts, but I wondered how the practice had been transformed for women. Arun didn't say, and I assumed that women could learn to control their energy, physical and sexual, in the same way as men.

"My masters used their body heat to live for a long time. They sat outside naked and melted the snow around them."

I could see them: lithe, muscular men—like Babaji—radiating heat. Slowly, I, too, was cultivating my inner fire through controlled breathing.

As I gained confidence in Arun, I told him about my misplaced trust in Chandra-swami and our ill-fated encounter. Instead of reprimanding me for my carelessness, he listened intently and responded with indignation. "The one thing I can't stand is men who hurt women and children. There is no worse crime for me. These people are cowards." Then he told me about Chandra-swami's known associations with the prime minister of India and other notable public figures. I had no idea he was so well connected.

While my private lessons progressed every morning, the entourage of female tourists continued to gather around Arun, and we often met up to chat in his room in the evenings. Chantal, a middle-aged French woman with shoulder-length blond curls, was the most outspoken and flirted openly with him. He told me privately that she had said, "Get that young girl away from you." Then he chuckled. "She thinks you're in love with me."

I shook my head. No one seemed to understand how an older man teaching a younger woman could be in a pure platonic relationship. He and I were close, but not in the way Chantal imagined. Arun had as little interest in sex with me as I had with James.

A few days later when I went up for my lesson at dawn, his eyes looked withdrawn. Once I was sitting down, he said, "Chantal slept here last night."

I shrank back at his unexpected revelation.

He looked into my eyes. "Nothing happened. She wanted to, but I didn't let it."

Why was he telling me this? And if he didn't want to be involved with her, why had he let her stay?

We moved on to the exercises for the day, but by evening I had no interest in the usual gathering. I lay on my bed: seething with jealousy, yet appalled at myself at the same time. Arun was more than thirty years older than me. How could I even think of him outside our teacher-student relationship? James was fifteen years older than me, already too old, and here I was developing feelings for a much older man. Worst of all my spiritual instructor. I was violating the purity of our relationship and the sacred teachings. Perhaps this was the hate he had warned about: the challenge I would need to overcome before the gift of immortality.

By the next morning, my mind had settled.

"Why didn't you join us last night?" Arun asked when I arrived for my lesson.

"I was tired. I wanted to rest."

He didn't say anything more but looked at me with care.

Later while I was having lunch in the reception area, I sat at a distance while he spoke with Chantal and her friend. My gaze took in his eyes: the brown irises dull and empty, they struck me as the eyes of a dead man. *Strange for a yogi.*

After Chantal and her friend had left the guest house to continue their travels, Arun showed me the blown-up prints of two portraits she had taken of him. In one, he was gazing at the river tenderly in profile; in the other he looked at the camera head-on with a boyish smile, challenging life to play along. She had captured two beautiful moments, and he was proud of the photos.

One evening, we sat side by side on the veranda outside his room watching a handful of lights speckled on the further bank. A breeze rustled over the invisible river below. He sat with his knees bent, feet up on the chair, his back curved grace-fully, and interrupted the quiet. "Have you ever been in love?"

I thought about it for a moment. "I don't think so."

"What about James?"

"No, definitely not James."

He pointed to his head. "You can think you're in love with someone, but that's just logic." Then he pressed the flat of his hand to his chest. "Or you can feel love in your heart. That's known as emotional pressure. But when you really fall in love, it's from here." He indicated his midriff. "Your belly won't lie to you."

I hadn't felt that unmissable jolt of love, but someday it would come my way: I was sure of it.

Gazing out into the darkness, he said, "People think they fall in love with the body, but it's the soul they fall in love with."

THE FORMAL YOGA course at the Forest Academy took place in a cement building up in the hills in a classroom that smelled of old paper. Rows of low desks were filled with white-pajamaed Indian male students. Two desks had been set aside for Julia and me, close to the door, across a corridor of space from the others. A young man with a boyish European face sat directly across from me. His head was shaved, and he wore the same plain attire as the others. He introduced himself by his Hindu name, Haridas. After we learned that we were both from New York, he quickly turned back to the male side of the room. I understood he was following the rules and didn't want to pursue further conversation.

Over the course of a morning, different professors came into the classroom and covered various facets of Hindu philosophy and religion. Yoga was presented as one of the major Indian philosophical systems, according to which matter and spirit can never be bridged. Yoga stands in opposition to Vedanta, which postulates the complete unity of spirit, mind, and matter in the universe.

Unaccustomed to sitting for hours with no backrest, I kept shifting my position to relieve the dull ache that gripped the base of my spine.

Twice a week, we practiced yoga poses in the early morning on the flat roof of the school building. A skinny male instructor called out Sanskrit words while we performed the poses on coarse wool blankets smelling of sheep. The wind whipped through the hills and permeated the thin fabric of my Indian pajama suit. Apart from the cold, the instruction felt arbitrary and impersonal, so unlike the dynamic stretches and strengthening exercises I was learning with Arun.

Since I had started my course at the academy, he had moved my instruction to lunchtime. One afternoon, our conversation turned to Babaji. Perhaps I had mentioned his feat of physical longevity.

"He was my master."

My jaw dropped, and I stared at him for a moment. "You mean *the* Babaji."

"Yes."

"The one who lived for centuries in the same body?"

He kept his eyes on me and nodded without a word.

His admission was so astonishing I couldn't take it in at first. Despite the many extraordinary claims made about yoga practice, it was mind-boggling for someone to know Babaji personally. Even more so, to have this person sitting right in front of me in the modest Ganges Guest House in Rishikesh. "I thought your master was Chinese."

"He was. Baba came from China. There he's known as Peng-tzu, master Peng."

Babaji was the apotheosis of the yogic pantheon, the only man who had defied death. There were even claims in New Age literature that Jesus Christ had been his student in the "lost years" before the events recounted in the gospels. "You know James was looking for Babaji?"

He shook his head. "Yeah, he told me. But why did he go to Badrinath?"

"I don't know."

"You won't find Baba there." He sighed. "He hasn't been seen for a long time."

Baba. He spoke of the divine master with loving familiarity, and a hint of sadness. I wondered what had happened to him, where he had gone.

Over the following days, Arun's teaching took on a deeper

meaning. I wasn't learning just any secret practice, but the authentic spiritual path mentioned in all the texts. No wonder James had felt particularly drawn to him. He was as close to enlightened as anyone could be on earth.

ONE AFTERNOON, when I returned from the Forest Academy, Arun was gone. His room was empty, and there was no sign of him downstairs. A knot of anguish formed in my belly, but soon Surat, Arun's young protégé, arrived and told me to come with him. He was a young lawyer starting out in his career, trying to make ends meet by defending criminals who weren't good payers. Arun saw an opportunity and took him under his wing. Surat took me on his motorcycle to Arun's new residence, an independent bungalow in an ashram in the hills.

The Swiss manager at the Ganges Guest House had insisted for some time that Arun attend her husband's evening lectures, and although Arun had resisted (as a swami he didn't need spiritual talks), she didn't agree and after he refused several times, she asked him to leave. His new residence—with its spacious living room, small kitchen, and bedroom—was a step up from a room at the guest house, and he showed me around with a satisfied smile. He had even employed a servant called Bahadur who would clean the bungalow, wash his clothes, and cook his meals. My daily lessons would continue at noon, followed by a home-cooked meal. It was the perfect arrangement for my student lifestyle.

I practiced on the hard tiles of the empty living room. The physical exercises had expanded to squats and abdominal conditioning, and he continued to watch me closely and adapt his teaching to my ability and development. After a month of the bamboo pole stretches, I could sit through the whole morning at the Academy without back pain.

One afternoon, Bahadur served a tray of *mooli paratha,* fried whole wheat flatbreads stuffed with white radish. I couldn't wait to break off a piece of the hot bread and dip into the red chili sauce, and waited for plates, but he didn't bring any. When Arun started to eat, I followed: hovering over the tray, taking pieces from the opposite side of the same bread. Eating from the same plate felt intimate, and it struck me that we weren't meeting for the first time. I felt so comfortable near him— drawn to his presence—we must have been close in a prior life. Probably lovers.

The idea of being born again wasn't new to me. In both the New Age and Hindu texts I had read, reincarnation is twinned with spiritual evolution: the soul, learning from past mistakes, grows in spiritual knowledge across multiple lifetimes. Reincarnation can explain not only varying life circumstances based on former good or bad deeds, but also different personal tendencies and aspirations. Mom thought of herself as an "old soul," seasoned from lifetimes of learning. She considered me in the same vein, well-traveled on the path of spiritual evolution. For as long as I could remember, praying since the age of three, I had felt the tug of spiritual experience. Later I developed a desire to understand my purpose on earth. Now destiny had brought me in contact with Arun.

When we were done eating, he leaned back and took a sip of Coke from his glass bottle. "There's a sexual aspect to the process. I would teach you if you were older." He paused. "At least thirty-five." He sounded like a clinician describing a routine process.

I wasn't surprised to hear that authentic yoga had a sexual component, but relieved that I wouldn't need to think about it for a long time. Thirty-five was an eternity away. Who knew where I would be by then and what I would be doing?

He dropped his tone. "I've only taught one other person. A woman I knew. She got close. But it didn't complete."

"What happened?"

"She died in a car crash."

"Oh, I'm sorry." He had told me about the many women who had been his lovers in California, but not this one. Had she been a client?

"It's bad when the process doesn't complete." He stopped and left it at that.

What was the implication of death with only partial spiritual knowledge? Or was he hinting perhaps that I had been this woman, returning now to complete my training?

I asked him what year she had died, then realized I couldn't be her; I had already been born by then.

I took a sip of Coke, appeasing the burn on my tongue with the syrupy liquid, and pondered my fate. I might not be the woman in Arun's story, but she was a kindred spirit. Like her, I was learning for a specific spiritual purpose.

He pressed the play button on his portable tape player, and Kenny Rogers' husky voice penetrated the room. He whispered along the words to "Lady," his favorite song, and I wondered who he was thinking about.

In his own space he was free and expansive. Far from keeping us apart, his move drew us closer together.

JULIA and I left the Academy together at the end of classes each day and walked down the hill. She dropped me off where Arun was staying, then continued to her own ashram. If it weren't for my lessons with him, I would have enjoyed having lunch and spending time together with her in the afternoon. The October temperatures felt like a Mediterranean summer, and as we ambled down the dirt path in companionable silence, the sun enveloped us in gentle warmth and enlivening light.

One day she asked, "You like him, don't you?"

My eyes widened at her suggestion. "Oh no, not like that."

Her mouth stretched into a smile, as if she could see something I hadn't admitted yet.

Inside, I shook my head: there was no romantic spark between Arun and me, no sexual tension polluting our relationship; our bond was pure.

I had changed so much already. I felt confident in the physical exercises, grounded in the daily energetic breathing. It felt like entering a different space, carried by the hypnotic rhythm of circular inhales and exhales. Deep within, I sensed the spiritual world Arun spoke of; in my body, the sought-after heat emerged.

He had spoken of further learning and the handful of students (men, I imagined) who had paid a fee of ten thousand dollars for the full course. "I call it the process of creative intelligence. It might sound expensive, but those who complete it are never the same again. Their lives are transformed physically, mentally, and emotionally."

He asked if I too wanted to learn the whole course, everything he knew, for eight thousand dollars. This time his request for payment didn't catch me off-guard, but it was a decision point. Did I want to stop or go further and deeper into the practice?

"You have been worshipping my master for a long time, that is why you have come to me," he said.

I had been tested and found worthy.

I knew from experience with TM and the Siddhis course that spiritual knowledge could be expensive, and that it was acceptable for a master to ask for something in exchange for years of accumulated experience. Eight thousand dollars was a lot of money, but I was on the brink of a new world. Baba guarded the gate, Arun held the key, and I was willing to take the leap.

I'd been exposed to wealth and what money can buy from an

early age. I was one of two girls in my class in Paris who had a governess and was aware that Maselle had been hired for my upbringing. In New York, I was the only girl whose driver brought her to school, and embarrassed, I'd ask him to drop me off a block away so I could pretend I had traveled on my own. When I turned twelve, I made a scene until Mom relented and allowed me to take the public bus. Both of my parents, whether individually or together, were absorbed in an extravagant lifestyle that I found confusing and alienating. But by my early teens, I focused on idealistic social pursuits and academic achievement.

Thanks to my parents' gifts since I had turned eighteen, I had money to pay Arun. I was saving it for my future, but here in the hills of Rishikesh, I had found what I longed for: a peaceful lifestyle coupled with spiritual study. Still, I didn't want to go ahead with the advanced course without letting them know. I called Dad and found out he would spend a couple of days in Delhi in November on his way to China. I would be done with my academy course by then and would tell him in person. There was no need to consult with James this time. So much had happened since he left; his presence felt like a distant memory.

Arun asked what I would do after my course. I didn't have much of a plan, but I wanted to visit the social activist Baba Amte. I had met him the year before during my thesis research in Central India when he had welcomed James and me into his home. Baba Amte came from a wealthy family and had started his career as a lawyer before Indian independence. He then gave up a lucrative practice to dedicate his life to caring for lepers, founding a charity for this purpose. He spoke to us about his work and life philosophy, and fed us a delicious meal served on banana leaves. He could no longer sit because of a back injury and ate standing up. His powerful presence and intelligence combined with his modesty and simple lifestyle left a lasting impression on me, and I wanted to ask him questions about his life choices and ethos.

I told Arun about him.

"I could travel with you if you want."

"You would do that?"

"Sure, if you want to. I could keep teaching you at the same time."

My eyes opened wide at his offer of companionship. I had been worried about how I would cope as a single woman without James, and now the universe was providing.

"You should see the south. That's the real India. The north is influenced by the Middle East."

"But I want to visit Baba Amte."

"We'll do that."

He sounded confident and offered to throw a party for me for my graduation. He asked me to invite Julia and Haridas, and I was touched by his thoughtfulness, delighted at the opportunity to introduce my master yogi to my classmates.

On the day of my graduation, we stood together at the back of the classroom. Swami Chidananda, the illustrious holy man whose shoulder Arun had healed, led the ceremony from the raised platform at the front. Sitting cross-legged with his long straight spine and emaciated frame, he surveyed the roomful of students with a solemn and kind expression. Arun had told me that despite their initial closeness, their relationship had faltered. Other swamis from the ashram had reported to him that Arun had appropriated a cave in Gangotri—a holy site high up in the Himalayas close to the mouth of the Ganges. "It was pure jealousy, but he listened to his people and didn't hear my side of the story." I had attended one of Chidananda's lectures in the past and found him aloof and distant, but today he took a presiding role. He was unaware of Arun in the audience and unfurled the scroll to announce the top students. I had studied for the exams without pressure and didn't know we would be ranked.

"In first place, Joelle Tamraz."

I was stunned to hear my name and walked up to the podium in front of all the men. Chidananda smiled and placed a garland of fresh marigolds around my neck.

In second place, he called Haridas.

I was proud that Arun had witnessed my unexpected honor and felt even more deserving of the lunch celebration he had planned.

After the ceremony, we walked down the hill together, and when we reached his bungalow, it was dark and empty. "Where's Bahadur?" I asked.

"He's visiting his family for a few days."

"What about the party?"

"What party?"

"For my graduation. You asked me to invite Julia and Haridas."

"It was today?"

I fought to hide my dismay. How could he have forgotten the date? He paused for a moment, as if expecting me to call it off, but I held his gaze. Our guests would be here any minute. Finally he said, "Let me find my wallet. I'll go buy some food."

Julia and Haridas arrived while he was still out, and just as we ran out of things to talk about, he returned with the food. It was already cooling, and the dishes were salty, but we ate out of hunger.

Haridas left shortly after the meal, but Julia stayed, and we chatted about our travel plans. She wanted to go to the south in search of a man she had once loved. They had separated when his parents forbade his marriage to a foreigner. I would be heading in the same direction with Arun. Before leaving she gave me a book of *Upanishads*, didactic "forest stories" from the Indian Vedanta tradition. She had written her name along with the Om symbol on the title page. I was touched by her gesture and wished I had thought of something for her.

When we hugged goodbye, her eyes filled with tears, and for a moment, I imagined a different outcome—one in which we had decided to travel together, rather than chasing our individual dreams.

6

LOVE IN PARADISE

We set off for our travels with Surat and his wife Usha. Arun had suggested the arrangement, and though I would have preferred to be alone with him, I understood it wouldn't be appropriate for an unmarried man and woman to travel together on their own. I had instructed my bank in New York to send the funds for the advanced course to Arun's newly opened account in Delhi, and as soon as we arrived, he withdrew the full amount in cash and stuffed it into a duffle bag. Back in his hotel room, he placed towers of stapled bills on his bed, lounged by the display, and invited Surat and Usha to join him. With a pack of bills held up across his chest, he greeted the camera with a straight face while Surat smiled and fanned another. In the image I captured, the three of them looked like unlikely robbers. As he repacked the bills in the bag, Arun said, "There's nothing dirtier than money."

Eight thousand dollars had materialized into a lot of rupees.

The four of us had gone on day trips together, and I enjoyed the company of my new friends. Surat and Usha were young

and in love, and they balanced Arun's mystique with their innocence. I was proud to fund the next leg of our journey, if
surprised at Arun's enjoyment of the physical cash.

When Dad arrived, I moved into the business hotel I had
booked for him near Connaught Place in the center of the city. I
knew from experience that time with him would be counted.
Even in my last year in Paris before moving to New York, when
I lived alone with my governess Maselle at the age of nine, he
had only come to see me a few times. He arrived long past my
bedtime, woke me up, and brought me to his room for a while.
Mom had gotten pregnant in the US and stayed in New York as
she was forbidden to travel by plane. I had returned to Paris for
the school year, and it would have been Dad's chance to spend
time with me. But of course, he didn't: that wasn't how he
worked. On the evenings he did show up, I didn't see him the
following morning, and by the time I was back from school he
was gone. I was so used to his sporadic presence and the
mystery that surrounded his movements that it didn't even
occur to me to wonder about it. When I moved to New York
that April to be with Mom and my new sister, Dad didn't join
us. My parents separated a couple of years later and divorced
five years after that, shortly after Dad's failed run for the
Lebanese presidency. He married Lena a year later.

Until he announced his visit to Delhi over the phone, I
hadn't believed he would actually come to India. He wore dress
trousers and a blue shirt with thick white stripes, the collar
open. He put on a carefree smile as we made our way around
Old Delhi, then walked around the colonnade of shops at
Connaught Place. Arun in his salmon outfit guided him like a
confident host. Dad stepped into an art gallery and came out
with four rolled-up prints from a famous Indian artist. He
placed the cardboard tube on his head in jest, and Arun's face
lit in a broad smile.

By his second day, Dad said we should go ahead without

him: he had things to do. I thought he had come to India to see me and was surprised by this sudden alternative agenda, but I didn't comment and joined my friends. When Dad and I met in our hotel room later that afternoon, he spoke excitedly about his day at one of the most opulent hotels in Delhi, raving about the lavish decor, the extensive buffet, and the high-class clientele. "Why didn't you book us a room there?" He looked at me questioningly.

I didn't have an answer for him. Since his career ended in Lebanon six years earlier—and his fortune went with it—he had spoken of various energy projects, but none had come to fruition so far. I wouldn't have considered such a luxury hotel. And why was he so excited anyway? The Park Hotel where we were staying was modern and comfortable. What had he discovered in the glass and marble palace? What else did he want to accomplish in India, apart from seeing me?

As Dad lay on his bed reading the day's newspaper, I collapsed on the other side in a sudden rush of choking feelings. There was no sound other than the occasional flick of a page, but my belly twisted as if I were at the top of a rollercoaster before the plunge. My breathing became shallow, and an uncontrollable urge to leave the room seized me. Yet I couldn't move: my body was pinned to the bed. The desire to run away from Dad was sudden and powerful, but I forced myself to reason through my panic. The rollercoaster would stop, and I would be on firm ground again; I just didn't know when. With each passing moment I felt more paralyzed, suffocating on my own energy.

It had been a long time since I had felt such overwhelming anguish. Most notably in childhood when Mom went to live next door after Saby's birth, I would lock myself in the small bathroom I shared with my sister and give in to loud, choking sobs. Mom was happy—an independent woman with new friends and a captivating boyfriend in a vibrant city—but how did I fit in? No one came to check on me during these fits. Letty, Saby's nanny, and the maid probably heard me, but they left me alone. I was grateful not to have to explain what was happening: because I had no idea. I had no words for my pain.

When I met Arun the following day, I told him about my disconcerting experience with Dad, expecting him to downplay, or even ridicule, the mental vortex in which I had descended. But to my surprise he was unfazed.

"You should have called me. I could have helped you. Next time it happens call me."

How simple. The day before I had felt stuck, helpless against the oppressive sensation. Now I had someone who cared.

WHEN I REVEALED to Dad how much I was paying Arun for his complete course, he didn't say anything, and I took his silence as acceptance. He had seen Arun for himself and understood my choice. Still, I was glad to have told him and not make a major decision behind his back.

On his third and last day in Delhi, we went for lunch at a fancy restaurant on Connaught Place. While we waited for our food, Arun leaned back and said to him, "Your daughter is a diamond in the rough. Carve her well," and smiled as if he had unearthed the diamond himself.

Dad wasn't one to praise and met Arun's effulgence with a passive expression, wondering, perhaps, at this man's glee.

On the morning of his departure, he handed me a white cardboard envelope. I opened it and found four round-trip plane tickets from Delhi to Chennai. His unexpected thoughtfulness and generosity astounded me.

"I didn't want you to spend so long on a train." He squeezed my shoulder. 'See you in New York."

After Dad left, I moved into the same hotel as the others, a more modest establishment in a bustling area of the city. When I told Arun about Dad's gift, he immediately suggested we exchange the tickets for cash.

"No. I want to go by plane."

There was no way I would give up Dad's gift and spend two days on a train with no shower or private toilet. I stood up to Arun for the first time, and after looking at me for a moment, he said nothing more.

The night before our flight to Chennai, I stayed in his room for a while after Surat and Usha had retired to theirs. He sat on his bed across from me with his legs bent and arms resting on his knees. The bedside lamp emitted a warm glow, and he looked at me with a somber expression.

"There is something I need to tell you."

I waited in the enveloping darkness.

"I've been alive for a very long time. One hundred and eighty years."

I stared at him for a moment, my lips parted. "In the same body?"

"I lost my original body. Arun was a very poor man. He could never feed his family. He had a bad heart, and I pushed him out." He looked at me, searching my expression.

I tried to make sense of his words.

"He left behind five children. He would have died anyway, but I gave the final push. It was wrong. I am indebted to his wife and children for the rest of my life."

I imagined the original Arun, weak and unable to make ends meet, then a spirit crossing from the other side, hovering over him, squelching his life, merging with his body. Who was the Arun I had met?

"He always wanted to be an actor." He shook his head in amusement. "But he could never make it." Then his eyes opened wide. "When I came back to India, I lived with his wife for some time. She sees me, but she knows something is wrong.

49

I am not the man she married. She made me sleep on a bench in the kitchen, so I left."

When had the Arun I knew lost his original body? When had he taken over another man's? The timeline was obscure. What was his original name? Someday I would ask more questions, but not tonight. It was enough that he had shared his terrible transgression and told me of the debt he would always bear to the family.

I returned to my much smaller room, lay in bed, and watched the shadows on the wall. I felt no fear. I had lingering questions but sensed that this man needed me, too.

ON OUR FIRST night in Chennai, he and I shared a hotel room. I trusted him and didn't mind the arrangement, but when it was time to go to sleep, I felt awkward lying on the bed next to his. He pulled out a miniature computer and started to type. He was writing a book on Agni Yoga, the yoga of fire, a knowledge he would someday share with the world. I fell asleep to the sound of his fingertips on the keyboard.

The next day he ordered two cups of South Indian coffee, a sweet milky concoction. I had never drunk coffee before, and once I tasted the warm, bitter-caramel liquid, I wondered why it had taken me so long to discover this morning pleasure.

Our destination was Mahabalipuram, a beach town on the Bay of Bengal, and there we had separate rooms again in a simple guest house a short walk from the ocean. Miles of empty sand stretched out in front of the endless view. Arun was proud of his native country and could speak several of its languages, including some of the local Tamil. He was eager to introduce me the south.

We brought our bamboo poles to the beach, and he showed Surat how to stretch by planting a pole in the sand and gripping the other end with his fists, so the pole stretched up in a diagonal line. Then he gently extended his arms and let his back hang like a hammock while his toes remained in the sand. His arm muscles were taut, and his skin glistened in the sun. Despite his age, he beat us all in agility.

We left the beach after our morning exercises and walked into town. Palm fronds swayed in the wind as Indian women in bright colorful saris—ochre, magenta, emerald—ambled on our path. Lunch was a typical South Indian meal: a cone of rice on a steel tray encircled by small bowls of lentil and vegetable preparations. Each dish had its own complex and subtle flavors, and despite its spiciness, the food was light and digestible. The meal ended with cups of sweet local coffee. The resort town was so quiet compared to the sensory overload of the north, the people so composed, and the pace of life so gentle, that I felt I had landed in paradise.

In the evenings Arun and I sat on the veranda steps outside our rooms and took turns reading aloud under the fluorescent tube light. He had assigned two books for my complete course: *Yoga: Immortality and Freedom* by Mircea Eliade and *The Secret of the Golden Flower: A Chinese Book of Life*. Eliade had been a professor, and Arun praised his work for its unadulterated straightforward explanations. So many books on yoga, he felt, were polluted by the author's agenda and personal opinions and strayed from the original truth. Unlike these other writers, Eliade had communicated the true yoga. In his text I found the familiar practices and aims of concentration, breath control, prolonging human life, even semen-retention. He defined the goal of enlightenment as renunciation of desire, its aim as liberation from the pain of living. Reading his words confirmed what I already sensed: the ultimate value of the spiritual life over the social pursuits of wealth, physical beauty, and worldly success.

The Secret of the Golden Flower was a much older text, veiled in imagery and cryptic language. Arun asked me to stop reading whenever I came across anything I didn't understand; he would then decode its hidden meanings. One passage referred to a spiritual body emerging from the physical body through concentration on inner emptiness. I understood it to be the spirit that Arun had cultivated, and which he now used to travel to the other side and meet with the elders and Baba.

I had experienced leaving my body as a child while lying in bed and contemplating the darkness. Out of nowhere, a thumb-sized version of myself appeared on the dresser across the room and gazed at my inert body. My consciousness had moved across the room, but looking at my body from a distance was so unsettling that I broke the spell instantly and rushed back into my body.

In later childhood and adolescence, I had a similar, though slightly less disturbing experience when playing a mind trick. While sitting on one of many slow bus rides in the city, I moved my awareness outside my body, as if I were looking at a stranger. *Who is this girl?* My hand appeared like a foreign object. My hair just a body's red hair, not belonging to me any more than the tree down the street. I didn't linger long in this state of observation because, like the diminutive version of myself that looked at my body lying in bed, dissociating from physical experience was unmooring, its implications unsettling.

Arun must have mastered the fear of separating from his body and learned to travel at will, and perhaps I would do the same someday; but for now, I was satisfied with the tangible confirmation of my progress. As he had predicted, a small muscular knot had formed at my perineum.

After we had finished reading one evening, the night air still warm, he got up, and as he walked to his room, he turned back, and the words "Good night, love" escaped from his mouth. He spoke so softly I almost didn't hear him, but he had said it. He was my teacher, and I felt love for him, but could it be the same for him? Did he love me, too?

On our last evening by the ocean, we went to a restaurant for dinner. Arun believed in eating a single main meal per day at lunch, and our dinners had consisted of savory South Indian snacks from the local street vendor. But he wanted to do something special before we left. We squeezed into tight seats around a rectangular table, and as he passed my chair to reach his, the hard pressure of his pelvis grazed my arm.

While we waited for our food, Surat and Usha smiled. Although they spoke little English, we communicated through facial expressions and a handful of words.

Arun spoke about the elders. "They have a mission for me. One morning millions of people will wake up from the same dream and recognize my face."

This seemingly messianic mission alarmed me. Even if it was necessary for the world, I didn't like the idea of millions of people recognizing my teacher as their spiritual leader.

"I told them I won't do it. Find someone else."

He sounded determined, and I relaxed. But it was the first time I understood the reach of the elders and the power of their plans. If they saw Arun as a savior, how long could he resist? There was still so much I didn't understand.

Our return journey took us through Mysore, where we visited the royal gardens and palace, and Bangalore, a larger more commercial city where we stopped at a mall. Arun asked Usha and me to pick out new Indian ladies' suits. I changed out of the male pajamas in which I felt comfortable and chose a white outfit with a fuchsia floral pattern down the middle. I left the shop in the starched tunic and trousers, a long matching scarf over my shoulder. With my hair braided down my back and gold hoop earrings, I felt confident in my new femininity and smiled with self-assurance in the photos he took on that day.

Back in Delhi at the end of our southern tour, he asked whether I wanted to replace my thick glasses. I hadn't given much thought to them before, but once he suggested the idea, it made perfect sense. We went to a gleaming optometrist on Connaught Place, and I selected designer frames with ultra-thin lenses. Since I'd sent the money from New York, Arun was paying not only for our trip to the south but also for the new suits, and now glasses. He wasn't just teaching me the secret practice, he was helping me become my best self.

7

IN LOVE WITH A YOGI

A few days before my flight to New York, I sat in my hotel room overlooking drab cement buildings with small windows and tangled electrical wiring. As I looked down at the knot of traffic below and listened to the muted sounds of vehicles honking, I realized that we hadn't stopped to visit Baba Amte on our way back, as I had intended. The thousand-kilometer journey west would have required planning, but I had left the itinerary in Arun's hands and followed his momentum. Perhaps I should have insisted that we go there; but at the same time, I felt so different from the new graduate who had arrived in India four months earlier. Stronger and more confident from Arun's exercise regimen and makeover, I had a plan for my life.

Before we left Rishikesh to travel, he had asked me to select a Hindu deity as the object of my prayers, and I hadn't hesitated to pick Shiva, lord of yoga and divine lover of the goddess Parvati. He symbolized two supreme aspects in one: enlightened freedom and unbreakable bond. He was also known as the god of destruction in Hinduism's three-fold notion of divinity as creation, upholding, and destruction, but it was his eternal connection with the goddess that spoke to me most clearly. Someday I would have the same relationship with my soul mate.

Sitting outside his bungalow in the hills, Arun had given me the standard Shiva mantra, *Om Namah Shivaya,* to repeat as often as I remembered. He had placed his right hand on my head in blessing, then said, "Now you bless me."

I raised my right hand as he had done, but he stopped me. "No, use your left hand. Women should bless with their left hand."

He bowed his head, and I placed my left hand on it.

Then he sat back and looked at me. "You were born to command, to control, and to serve."

Another prophecy. I wasn't sure about the first two elements, but service felt natural. I had told him I wanted to be a social activist, but he had advised me to make my own money before trying to help others.

With his guidance, I was taking the right step, at the right time.

I went to sit on the bed for my morning meditation and tucked my left heel under my pelvis. I bent my head, drew my chin to my chest, and let silence take over the darkened inner space. With each controlled breath, I grew more distant from the world, abandoning my social persona, and dwelling in a cocoon of inner vibrations. I stayed in place twenty minutes, maybe more, and when I lifted my head and released my heel, tears streamed down my face. In that quiet space I had sensed the presence of Babaji, maybe even God. This deep connection only happened rarely; but when it did, it was powerful.

Suddenly I couldn't imagine an abrupt end to my time with Arun, a return to my former life in New York as if nothing had happened. The secret practice was revelatory, and I was on the cusp of a new state. I couldn't leave it all behind.

That same evening I knocked on the door of his room, and

he invited me in. He sat cross-legged in his orange pajama suit and matching wool sweater, leaning against the pillows of the single bed. His face bloomed into a luminous smile when he saw me, and he called me by the nickname he had invented. "Jewel, sit."

I placed myself at the edge of his bed, looked away, and blurted out the words I had come to say before I lost my nerve.

"I've been lying to you. I'm not just your student. I love you."

I waited for his displeasure at the betrayal of our sacred relationship, but his face remained calm, his expression gentle. Then he spoke in slow measured tones. "I know. I love you too. You are my wife. You have been chosen for me."

The word "wife" melted my anguish and revealed why I felt so close to him despite our age gap.

"When I met you, I had been planning to stay in my cave for the winter. I had bought all the supplies. But then the elders told me you were there, and I had to come down and find you."

I listened in rapt silence.

"I didn't believe them at first. I thought they were tricking me. But then they showed me your picture." He smiled. "I told them you look skinny, but they said I should fatten you up."

He held out his thick hands toward me, and I touched his palms, warm and soft. "You are my wife returned to me."

"How long? How long have we been apart?"

"A very long time."

Light radiated from his face and enlivened his eyes. I moved in closer and smelled the Dove soap on his skin. Then gently I placed my lips on his. They felt thin, frailer, and older than I expected, but his arms wrapped around me, and I felt safe.

After a moment I pulled back from him slightly and contemplated his face. Its golden sheen made him look androgynous. "Your face. It's different."

"It's my night face. When the elders are here."

I looked around, suddenly self-conscious. "Are they here now?"

"Yes, they wanted to see you. But don't worry. They'll leave us alone."

I returned to my room to change, and when I joined him again, he opened the sheets for me to lie with him. He wanted to make love, but I couldn't; not right away, not so soon. He still felt like my teacher, and we slept snuggled in the single bed, but when we stirred around midnight, we made love then, for a few minutes, and he apologized for the briefness of our encounter. "It's been so long since I've been with a woman."

I didn't care. I hadn't come to him for sex, but for love. The love beyond time and space I had anticipated my whole life.

I awoke the next morning as light filtered through the curtains; still nestled in his body, his hand resting on mine, for a moment I couldn't tell where I ended and he began.

8

INTERLUDE

I sat on the wool carpet and looked down at Fifth Avenue from the 39th floor of Mom's apartment. Close to Christmas, the avenue was a lit belt of matchbox cars, the pavement filled with people scurrying in every direction with their work bags and packages, pushing to get ahead. Where were they all going? After spending months in India, mostly in small towns, I felt out of tune with this purposeful drive.

I was back in the place where I had grown up since the age of nine; where I had lived in the master bedroom sandwiched between Saby and Letty who slept in the second bedroom and Mom in the apartment next door. At first I was overwhelmed by all the changes: the sudden rupture of my life in Paris—there had been no time to say goodbye to Maselle or my closest friend—my new sister, and a vastly different country, culture, and school system. I waited years for Mom to open a passage between the apartments and merge our separate lives. But by the time I became a teenager and our living arrangement had remained intact, I was used to my independence. I had a huge room to myself and focused on my studies and after-school work at the Junior Academy of

Sciences. When I left for college, Mom returned to the family home, took over the master bedroom, and rented the apartment next door. The days of rupture were long gone. Unspoken and buried.

When Saby and I were younger, Mom invited friends to spend Christmas Eve with us. With no other relatives in New York, they were our chosen family, and the holidays felt full. But on my return from India, with Saby now thirteen and Letty retired a year earlier, it was just the three of us for Christmas. Something was missing, and already I longed to return to India and be with Arun.

Phone calls were expensive, and I didn't want to attract Mom's attention, but when I managed to speak with him I brought up a question that had been worrying me.

"What would have happened if I hadn't come to your room that night?"

"I would have let you go."

"And we would have never seen each other again?" I was shocked by how close we had come to losing each other again.

"The decision has to come from the woman. It doesn't work otherwise." Then he quickly added, "I knew you would come to me."

Arun thought the world of women. He had once told me that the only gods in the universe are women because they can deliver children. Another time he'd said, "I can drive any car," alluding to his sexual abilities.

After we hung up, I mulled over his words. How could he simply let me go, after the elders had informed him of my return? How could we have separated after our reunion? We had found each other again, declared our love to each other, but surely it couldn't stop there.

I decided to postpone the start of my consulting job and use the rest of my grant money to return to India for the rest of the year. Life after university felt like an achievement train, and I wasn't ready to jump on it. I was a dreamer and had other plans.

When I told Mom about continuing my travels, she moved her reading glasses up to her head. "Aren't you done with India now?"

"Not yet. I want to learn more from the teacher I met there."

She thought for a moment. "Well, if you plan to go back, I'll take Saby and we'll come to visit you during her vacation in February."

I got in touch with James to tell him I was home, and he asked why I hadn't returned any of his phone calls.

"What phone calls?"

"I called you many times and left you messages. Surat said he would pass them on."

I had given him Surat's landline number, but he hadn't mentioned any calls. There was no reason for him to withhold James's messages unless he had instructions to do so. Maybe Arun had wanted to shelter me from past influences during my critical learning period.

James continued to speak in his breathy cloying voice, and I hurried to end the call. I knew I would never speak to him again.

A friend from university came over for a visit, and after we had been chatting for a while, she said, "You've changed. It's like you take up more space now."

Arun had warned me not to tell anyone about the secret practice, but rather let people notice the change for themselves. I hadn't seen this friend since graduation, and her observation validated his prediction: my training had given me a presence and confidence I lacked at university.

I needed bamboo poles to continue my stretching exercises and enlisted Dad's help to go to a lumberyard downtown. We bought pine rods, the closest equivalent we could find. Although Arun had prohibited me from teaching the secret practice, I shared the physical exercises with Mom and showed her how to perform spinal side stretches and twists.

When he and I spoke again, he asked me to send him the American clothes he missed. I offered to bring them with me at the end of January, but he wanted them sent by courier. He didn't specify what to buy so I chose jeans, t-shirts, sweatshirts, sweatpants, and a cashmere sweater as a special gift from me. I packed all the items in a large cardboard box and called an international courier to pick it up. The cost of shipment exceeded the price of the goods. Arun's insistence felt extravagant, but I didn't want to clamp down on his enthusiasm.

Over dinner with the same friend from university, I recounted his request and the high cost of shipment, then caught myself. How could I already be speaking behind his back? He had said people who complain about their partners aren't really in love, those relationships are already broken. They might not end immediately, but sometime, somewhere, they would. I vowed to be more careful in the future.

He had also told me that the secret practice couldn't be found in books; it had been handed down from teacher to student over centuries. Still, I made my customary pilgrimage to Borders bookstore on Park Avenue and headed straight to the eastern religion shelves. I couldn't find any references to inner fire or immortality in the Buddhism titles, but in the books on Taoism, it was all there: the root fire, the cauldron or solar plexus, stoking the fire or breathing for physical longevity. I bought a couple of them.

In *Taoism: The Road to Immortality*, I read a story that the author claimed was true. A scholar abandoned his life in the city and set off into the mountains in search of spiritual knowledge. There he met an immortal called Hulu-wang (Gourd Immortal) who described his teaching in such colorful language that the scholar thought he had made a mistake and decided to leave in the morning. Then two young girls who attended to the immortal and were thought to be his grand-daughters went to speak with the scholar and persuaded him to stay. He undertook a long apprenticeship and became a divine master in his own right and ultimately the immortal's heir. This story captivated me. The scholar's journey from the city to the mountains, his interest in books, his initial apprehension followed by later success reminded me of my experience.

After a few weeks away from Arun—Saby had returned to school by then, and Mom to her demanding work as a clinical psychologist—the pain of separation felt acute. I awoke one morning with a vision of him sitting above my bed in the lotus pose in his usual salmon clothes, a radiant impassive expression on his face. His silent presence brought a sense of deep peace, as if he had projected himself to comfort me. From then on, I felt less alone.

9

ONE FOR THE OTHER

As I pushed my luggage cart through the airport gates, the earthy combination of dust and sweat rose to my nostrils. In the warmth of the Delhi night, I searched for Arun beyond the throng of beige-suited men crowding the gate and finally spotted him in the distance. He was leaning against the car, limbs limp at his side. His hair was grayer than I remembered, and he looked older. But as I approached and he caught sight of me, his face opened into a luminous smile, and my first fleeting impression was quickly replaced by the joy of reunion.

He had moved from Rishikesh to a penthouse in Delhi but didn't explain why. We had our own space in one of the most elegant neighborhoods of the capital, and I walked through the apartment with excitement, discovering his belongings as I went. Clothes piled in the wardrobe, toiletries scattered in the bathroom, books placed haphazardly on the living room shelf. I had never lived with a man before and took in the details as if I had entered a living museum. I slotted in my clothes among his, careful not to upset his whimsy, and resisted the urge to tidy up his belongings. I didn't want to disturb his tantalizing energy.

His servant Bahadur, who had joined him from Rishikesh, cleaned the place, cooked our meals, and washed Arun's clothes, but not mine. February sunshine was already persistent, the days balmy. I braved the cold water to wash my clothes, then hung them out to dry in the inner courtyard. Arun was happy to see me and took me to the nearby market, an assortment of expensive shops around a square. I bought the finest muslin suits—one warm yellow, the other pale green—and gave no thought to how our living was paid for. I basked in the certain joy of our new relationship.

He took the lead in bed, and I trusted him and felt content to discover what our love would reveal. At night he wore the gardenia perfume he had asked me to buy for him in New York, and I delighted in his definition of male attractiveness, so different from the typical American, or even European, male. With his pierced ears and growing curls, he combined the warmth and familiarity of Middle Eastern culture and the mystical allure of an Indian yogi.

It took two weeks for him to say, "You've finally opened up to me."

I was glad to have met his expectation of physical intimacy, though I didn't know he had been waiting. We fell asleep in each other's arms, and I awoke to the sound of the spinning fan. I didn't want to be anywhere else and could have stayed there forever.

But despite our closeness, I was still his student and practiced my breathing meditation religiously at the start of each day. One morning, when I was done, a question surfaced in my mind: *Why me?* Why had Arun chosen me over James to learn the secret practice? Surely James, who knew so much about yoga, would have been the better candidate. I don't know why the concern arose at that moment, but without further thought, I voiced it to Arun.

His face clouded over, and he stared into my eyes. "Why are you asking me this?"

I realized my mistake instantly, and my chest tightened. "No, I, I just wanted to know."

"Have you not understood anything I've been teaching you?"

I had witnessed the scenes he made in stores where he had bought an item and came back to mouth off about the quality, large hands pressed into the counter. Whoever was there listened, so sure was he of his own position, so certain of his demands. But he had never turned that intimidating voice on me. The change in his mood was so sudden I couldn't speak. I sat on the bed in silence.

He stood in front of me, unmoving. "Answer me."

"I . . . I don't know."

"If you asked, there must be a reason. I want to know."

The more he pressed, the less I could defend myself. I felt like a child. All I could manage through the knot in my throat was, "I'm sorry. I don't know what made me say it."

"Looks like I've made a bad mistake." He left the room with quick determined steps.

I dropped my head to the pillow and melted into sobs. How could I have thought of such a question when he had already told me he had chosen me specifically? What had made me bring up James? How had I ruined everything so soon? With each spiraling thought, I sank deeper into a dark well.

For a few minutes, I wallowed in the terrible situation I had created, unable to see a way out. Then he returned to the room, looked at me lying there, and held out his hand. "I'm sorry. I overreacted."

I ignored the pain in my head and sat up. I took hold of his hand, relieved that he was back so soon, though a little confused.

He pulled me up. "I shouldn't have spoken to you like that. I'm sorry. The elders reprimanded me."

Our first fight had taken me by storm, and I was still shaken by the chain of events. I steadied myself on the firmness of the floor and let him encircle me in his arms. "It's okay," I said.

The quickness of his recovery from ominous rage reminded me of how Maselle sometimes picked on something I had done and blew it out of proportion, her reaction explosive but short-lived. Her strongest threat against my misbehavior was to leave me outside the kitchen entrance of our apartment in Paris. She evoked the threat often but only acted on it once; I don't remember the reason. Once she had closed the door the stairwell was pitch black. But I didn't even have a chance to get used to the darkness before she opened it again. In that moment I realized her words were empty: she had no intention of leaving me there.

After apologizing, Arun led me into the living room and faced me square on. Then he held up his thumb and forefinger and rubbed them together until a faint stain, the color of rust, appeared. "The blood of the elders." He pressed his index finger between my eyebrows. "Nothing will be able to separate you from us now."

I went to look at myself in the bathroom mirror and saw a brownish spot on the legendary third eye. Perhaps it was to open my vision. But more importantly, it was our seal, and no force would be able to divide us.

When I returned to the living room, he said, "Let's go out."

"Where?"

"To the market. I want to show you something."

We reached the familiar square after a short autorickshaw ride, and he headed straight to the computer store, a modern space that smelled of electronic machines and the chill of air conditioning. I wandered between displays and lingered over laptops.

"Choose one."

I looked at a price tag and did a quick calculation. Two thousand dollars—more than we could afford. I told him so, but he was determined. "You need something to keep you busy."

I returned home with the latest slimmest laptop, placed it on the living room table, and opened Word. Arun looked on with a smile as I started to type into a document. Who was this man of many faces and changing moods? How did he understand my needs before I did?

The following morning, I aligned all the books on the shelf in descending order of size, then arranged his clothes into neat piles. The apartment no longer reflected his spontaneity, and already I missed his unbounded energy. But nothing could be done: my initial abandon had gone.

ARUN'S FAMILY, the one that came with the dying man's body, lived in Delhi. He had a particularly good relationship with one of his daughters. She was a few years older than me, and when he took me to her home, she and her husband welcomed me with warmth. Their maid served us tea on a tray in a dim curtained room. If the couple wondered about this young woman at their father's side, they didn't show it. The daughter couldn't have understood about the spirit in her father's body, but perhaps she accepted that he had left her mother and started a new relationship.

From my side, I didn't question his duties to this family and enjoyed the daily social call. Our visits provided a welcome break from the spiritual world that haunted Arun; regular family concerns and the real world replacing life-and-death spiritual duties. His daughter's acceptance of me also helped me to feel at home with him.

One night in a dream, I saw different colored dresses floating into the sky and heard Babaji say, "Changing bodies is like changing clothes." I took it as a lesson about the transmigration of souls and awoke with a firm sense of my rightful place in Arun's spiritual family. I shared everything with him and told him about the dream.

MOM AND SABY arrived later that month, and though I went to stay with them at The Park Hotel, I brought them to our apartment. After Mom had seen the place, she said, "There's only one bed here. The two of you are in a relationship."

I denied it immediately and pointed to the backless couch in the living room. "Arun sleeps here."

She kept quiet and didn't pry; or maybe she wanted to believe me.

Arun showed paternal interest in Saby and put her at ease. After a couple of days, she said, "I like him," and I trusted her unbiased instincts.

We took the family to Old Delhi and stopped at a traditional perfume shop with different scents in small glass vials. Mom chose authentic rose. Then we went to a jewelry shop, and Saby, who was almost fourteen, bought pieces she'd never seen before: an upper-arm cuff and a detailed waist chain, both of pure gold.

Mom seemed at ease in India. She commented on how the heat and the wooden carts heaped with fruits and vegetables reminded her of her childhood in Cairo when sellers called out from the street below and hoisted baskets of produce up to open windows.

While I was in New York, Arun had asked me to buy three gold coins. He believed all ancient cultures valued gold's healing and protective powers. He insisted on pure gold coins, the Chinese Panda or Canadian Maple Leaf, and I accepted the expense as a necessity. Finding them had taken time and persistence. He had the coins mounted and gave one to each of us, instructing us to wear them under our clothes, so the gold touched our skin.

After her initial question about our relationship, Mom showed acceptance toward Arun, and spoke with him in hushed tones. I didn't ask her about their discussions, but Arun later told me that she had confided in him about issues following her divorce. He had suggested that powerful prayers would improve her luck. All she had to do was write her wishes on individual pieces of paper and fold them. He would then take them to a reputable Brahmin family, and the traditional Hindu priests would pray day and night without pause for their realization. The ritual was expensive—seven thousand dollars —but the family was genuine, and their prayers effective.

I was surprised by Mom's private trust in Arun, though it reminded me of how she had taken James into her confidence. She wasn't inherently opposed to paying for spiritual guidance —from fortune-tellers to the advanced TM program—and if all seven wishes came true, as Arun promised they would, the money would soon be forgotten.

When Saby and Mom returned to New York, he asked me if I wanted to see her wishes.

I refused. Weren't the wishes supposed to remain secret? I was shocked that he would betray her trust after promising to commission prayers for her.

SOON AFTER, he announced that we were returning to Rishikesh; the landlady in Delhi was being unreasonable and they had had a fight. But before we left, I asked him when he would buy me bangles, the adornment I had seen on all Indian women. He smiled in surprise and later apologized to me for not thinking of it himself; the elders had reprimanded him for his missing this important step in our relationship. He took me to a trustworthy jeweler and asked me to select the design of my choice. I chose two solid gold circles in the shape of a snake biting its tails. I put one on each wrist and admired our shining link.

On the drive from Delhi to Rishikesh, Arun brought up my sister and commented on how lucky he was to have met two such intelligent young women, both of whom he could teach. His words made me bristle—Saby was too young to learn the secret practice, and in any case she had no interest in the spiritual world of the elders. He wouldn't be teaching her.

We moved into a small house in the hills with a breathtaking view over the Ganges valley below. Our landlord, who lived next door, was a well-known social activist. I would have taken more interest in his work if Arun hadn't focused my attention on the spiritual life.

I practiced every day and recorded my experiences of "blanking out" or seeing a clear blue light in my journal. Arun had told me, "The magic is in the extremes"—the moments when I either held my breath in or remained without air. Physical vibrations and sweating confirmed my progress. And when I lifted my head and opened my eyes from meditation, the world appeared renewed.

Whatever I reported to him from my meditations he deemed normal—natural results of the practice, like a car changing directions at the turn of a wheel. Longevity was the end result of a lifetime of discipline. Though I never saw him meditating, I imagined he had outgrown the daily work and could now escape from his body at will.

Our daily conversations bound us together, and I listened intently as he filled in the pieces of his story. He had lost his parents at the age of eight during the partition of India and been left in the care of an uncle who couldn't afford to raise him and took him to live with yogis in the Himalayas. He was vague about the location and reiterated that they had lived somewhere on the border of India and China, which could have been Tibet, Nepal, or indeed, India. As a young boy he resisted his new masters and kept trying to run away, but each time, they would uncover his hiding spot, as if by magic. In time, he accepted his new home and became Babaji's protégé, and eventually his designated heir.

He told me how the elders once found him sleeping under a tree while a king cobra raised its head before him, a sign of his exceptional spiritual destiny. It seemed astonishing, and I wondered where in the Himalayas king cobras lived.

In one of his sweetest stories, he recounted how Babaji, a man who had escaped all worldly attachments, became so enamored with Arun's childish whimsy and playfulness that he bestowed a blessing upon him: no matter how old he grew, he would always keep his childlike nature. Indeed, his spontaneous charm was still evident and infectious.

In the rising heat of the afternoon, we retired to the bedroom where I discovered pleasures of the body I attributed to our deepening love. I had never felt so close to anyone. In my long-term significant relationships in high school and university, something had always been missing. The intimate physical connection I felt with Arun had been absent. He believed that a man's pleasure should be subordinate to a woman's—even avoided. He was gentle and loving and made me want to stay with him endlessly. Our intimacy replaced the feeling of aloneness I had felt for so long.

I was lucky to have found him: lover, fawn, child.

It wasn't just physical closeness. In the late afternoon, we sat on the cot at the entrance of the house and watched the sunset blanket the hills as the day's heat relented slightly. He challenged me with questions and listened intently when I spoke.

One day he asked about my plans, and I said I didn't have any; I wanted to stay with him.

"You'll get bored here."

"I won't."

"What about working with your father?"

"My father? Why would I want to do that? He and I don't get along. He doesn't even remember our birthdays. Mom has to remind him."

"Who told you that? Your mother? Why don't you find out for yourself?"

I wasn't convinced.

His voice was gentle. "There's something called letting the inner child grow."

I asked him about the half-moon nail on the top joint of his thumb. He splayed his hands, thick fingers wide apart. "Nothing. I was born like this." Bending the top joint, he added, "These are special thumbs. If I hadn't followed the spiritual path, I would have been a criminal." He smiled.

Of course he wasn't a criminal.

A few days later, he encouraged me again to work with my father. "You go first. Once you're settled, bring me into the work."

At two-and-a-half months, my stay in India turned out to be shorter than I expected. I listened to Arun's counsel, and we took the drive back to Delhi. We went to eat pizzas at our favorite restaurant on Connaught Place before my flight, and when we'd finished eating, he sat back and looked at me directly. He had something to tell me: he had a promising business opportunity in Rishikesh; would I lend him thirty-thousand dollars? He raised an open palm. "I swear on Baba I'll pay you back. Someday you will forget about this money, but I won't. I will give it back in your hands."

Thirty-thousand dollars was the rest of my savings; if I lent it to him, I would be giving him everything.

We were joined body and soul; a loan felt awkward. "Why don't you make me your business partner? I'll invest with you." That way, I could justify the loan and share in the profits.

He reassured me. "No, no. Let me borrow it. It's better this way."

Husband in my past life, he would be again someday in this one—I had no doubt about it. I accepted his promise of repayment. There was nothing to fear.

10

CROSSFIRE

Arun sent me home with lavish gifts for my family: handwoven silk carpets from Kashmir for Mom, Saby, and Dad, and an antique cane with a stone-inlaid sheath for Dad. He had even bought me a royal-blue pure pashmina shawl. Everyone appreciated their gifts other than Lena, Dad's Lebanese wife, who sent the carpet for immediate fumigation.

When I told Dad I wanted to work with him, after an initial moment of surprise, he asked me to meet his Lebanese business associate, Elie, at their new midtown office. Elie greeted me with a firm handshake and a smile. He introduced me to the Caspian Sea gas projects they were working on and enlisted my help to draft business correspondence.

The office had two rooms connected by a passageway. Elie occupied the one at the back, and Claire—the office assistant, a pleasant South African woman in her mid-thirties—sat at the front. Several times an hour Elie bellowed her name from his office while she raised her eyebrows at me in silence. When she found out I would be working with them regularly, she was delighted.

I contacted the consulting firm in Cambridge and told them I would not join after all, then asked Claire to pay me a monthly stipend of two-thousand dollars: the equivalent of what I would have earned at the job, minus rent. With no savings and a long-distance relationship, I needed money.

Arun fed our love affair with long missives sent by fax. His words were testaments of his love; the emptiness he had felt before we met; and the unique place I now occupied in his life. He also spoke of my progress on the spiritual path. Never before had someone expressed so much longing for me.

I had taken back a cassette of Jagjit Singh's album *Insearch*, a series of languorous Urdu songs Arun played on repeat in Rishikesh. Although he asked me why I wanted to listen to songs whose words I couldn't understand, they reminded me of him and our life in India. They kept me connected with him while I transitioned to a completely different experience in New York.

He was adamant that I mustn't reveal our relationship to anyone—especially not my mother, who, he said, had taken a dislike to him based on her "feminine jealousy." The elders had revealed that she had fallen in love with him and would refuse to pay for her prayers if she found out he was in a romantic relationship with me.

In one of his letters he wrote, "We can do the work of BABA for the rest of our time. Any taint in this union will destroy the power we have got now . . . any weakness will destroy the hard work put into this union by the ELDERS."

Mom was a witness to the flow of daily faxes, but I made sure to retrieve the sheets of paper from her bedroom before she could pick them up. One evening the machine started its characteristic hiss, and I ran into her room as page after page of a particularly long letter flowed out. Mom was lying in bed reading, and Saby was doing her homework at her desk, typing on the computer. After I'd collected all the sheets, Mom removed her glasses and stared at me.

"That's not a relationship between a teacher and a student." I froze.

She kept observing me. "Sit down. I want to speak to you."

My heart tightened, and I sat at the edge of the green upholstered chair near her bed.

"What's going on?" she asked.

I avoided the pressure of her stare. "Nothing."

She waited, her eyes latched on to me, willing me to answer.

I buckled under the strain and blurted out, "We're together."

Fury filled her eyes instantly. "How could you? He's old enough to be your grandfather."

Saby stopped typing and looked up.

Arun was Dad's age; why did she have to exaggerate to make it seem worse? My throat constricted. I had nothing more to say to her and left the room and went straight to bed. I didn't know which was worse, betraying Arun's confidence or Mom's reaction. Later that night I felt Saby kiss my cheek. When I asked her about it the next morning, she said I had been crying in my sleep.

I ran into Mom as she was preparing to leave for work, and she stared me down, the intensity of her feelings unabated. "He's a bad, bad man. All he cares about is sex and money."

I was shocked by the strength of her reaction, the profound error in her judgment.

"If you're going to be with him, you can't stay here."

She left and shut the door behind her, and I called Dad. I told him what happened and how Mom had kicked me out of the house.

"You said you were just friends."

"I know, but something changed."

I asked if I could stay at his new apartment on the Upper East Side, and he agreed.

When I told Arun about my exchange with Mom, he was concerned. "She won't pay me now."

"She will. She won't go back on her promise."

THAT SUMMER, we met in Paris. He couldn't travel to the US—though he hadn't told me why—and I would keep working for Dad from his small Paris office. I rented an apartment for six weeks based on an internet listing—a new experience for me—and was relieved to find it was as nice as the few photos posted online.

Dad's side of the family was staying with Lena and him at their large Paris apartment: his sister, Mireille; Saby; and my younger siblings, Eduardo and Margherita, children of Dad's second partner before Lena. Eduardo was twelve and Margherita eleven, and they lived with their mother in Rome. I had only met them five years earlier; until then their existence had been kept secret from Saby and me. Mom didn't want us to know Dad had fathered other children while still married to her. It was only after I turned eighteen and Saby nine, that Dad organized a dinner to introduce us to our younger siblings, who were then seven and five—sweet children who held no responsibility for their parents' complicated lives.

But by then I already knew. I overheard Mom and Dad speaking about them two years earlier in the living room of our New York apartment. When I told my boyfriend about my incredible discovery, he confessed that he already knew—everyone in my parents' social circle did—and at sixteen, I felt embarrassed to have been in the dark for so long. When I finally met my siblings two years later, Dad had already been separated from their mother for some time and married Lena.

Arun and I visited the family every morning, and he led a

group stretching session in the open space of the living room. Eduardo and Margherita joined in and followed his engaging teaching style. We went out to dinner with my aunt, and she seemed to accept my charming companion. I was relieved that not everyone shared Mom's punishing opinion.

About three weeks into our trip, Arun said he needed to tell me something. We were sitting together in the living room after a long afternoon nap.

"You might not want to be with me after you hear this. I'll understand, but you need to know it."

I sat up straight and took a deep breath, confident that there was nothing he could say that would change my feelings for him.

After years of living in Los Angeles, he had moved north to the Napa Valley to escape from danger. He didn't specify what kind of danger, but I understood it to be spiritual, linked to his work on the other side. In the new town, he met a marijuana dealer who introduced him to two teenage girls. A few days later, the girls knocked on his door. They were drunk, skipping school, and asked him for a place to stay. He let them rest in his bedroom.

How could he have let them in? I already knew the end of the story.

They stayed for a while, and after they left, Arun forgot about them until a couple of weeks later, on Halloween night, the police knocked on his door, searched his house, and took him away in handcuffs.

"I tried to escape danger, but I walked right into it. I can still remember the cold metal on my skin. Up to now I hate Halloween."

"Why did you let them in?"

"I didn't do anything to those girls. Let them lie on my bed. That's it." His eyes opened wide. "That dealer framed me."

I shook my head.

"I didn't have money for my own lawyer. The state assigned a lawyer who knew nothing about this kind of case. He said I had to plead guilty. I didn't want to, but he said it might be different if I was white, but the jury would never believe a brown man."

I felt angry and upset for him, knowing how with the racism in my country, he wouldn't stand a chance.

He was given a five-year sentence, then released after three years. He thought his troubles were over, but before he could even find a permanent home, the Department of Immigration took him in. He chose deportation to India rather than remain in prison for an indefinite amount of time. When I met him in Rishikesh, he had been back a year.

"I want to go back. The US is my home. I want to fight this case."

This man who had been gentle and loving with me, who believed women were divine beings deserving of care and respect, would never hurt girls—I was sure of it. His pain was still fresh, and I set aside my dismay at his poor judgment: he had made one thoughtless mistake.

"I want to speak with your father. He needs to hear from me personally."

I arranged a meeting at Dad's customary cafe on the Champs Élysées, and when Arun returned, he said Dad had asked him for three promises: we wouldn't get married; we wouldn't have children; and I would apply for an MBA degree.

Shortly after his revelation, Arun was ready to leave. We still had two weeks of the six-week rental, and I was surprised he wanted to go so soon—especially as we didn't know when we would see each other again. But he wanted me to get to work and find a good lawyer to overturn his case. Dad had promised to help, and I was eager for Arun to join me in the US. Maybe it made sense not to waste time.

Before we separated, he said the elders had reprimanded

him for focusing more on sex than on teaching me while we were in Paris. He promised to do better next time.

As soon as I was back in New York, I ordered the case files and pored over reams of documents from the court reporters. The sexual acts he had supposedly committed were described in such detail that I wondered why the girls would take such pains to fabricate a story. I couldn't bear to linger on those pages and moved on quickly.

Then other statements made me pause. The police had found a single bottle of wine and hundreds of Lotto tickets in the kitchen—strange for a yogi who didn't drink. I dismissed these details as oddities and assumed he'd received the bottle of wine as a gift. And while I didn't believe in the value of playing the Lotto, it looked like he did.

A couple of incongruous facts would have been fine, but the next section stopped me cold: Arun had obtained his green card through marriage to a woman in California. There was no mention of divorce. I had been reading the files at Dad's office, but phoned Arun immediately. When I questioned his marriage, he sounded unperturbed.

"It was only for my green card. That marriage was annulled. She was already married."

"You never told me you were married."

"Did I not tell you?'"

"No, you didn't."

"If I had been married, they couldn't have deported me."

That was a point. His relaxed confidence eased my troubled mind. A hidden marriage was an enormity too difficult to contemplate. I dropped the matter, but the image of the lonely bottle of wine on the kitchen counter stayed in my mind.

Dad worked with a woman whose brother was a criminal lawyer, and he asked me to give her the files. After reading them, she concluded that the girls' accounts had been made up. What a relief: this mature woman vindicated my view. She passed on the documents to her brother, who reviewed the case and said it would be impossible to reverse. According to a recent change in immigration law, a resident alien convicted of aggravated felonies was barred from returning to the US, even if married to an American citizen. The lawyer delivered his assessment over the phone in a gentle tone and ended with an off-the-record suggestion: Arun could change his name.

But he didn't like this outcome. He wanted his name cleared, not a return under false pretenses. Besides, a fingerprint check would link him to his past, and he wouldn't survive a second bout in prison.

At the same time as I oversaw the investigation, I worked with Elie on Dad's gas projects and managed the logistics to host a symposium of over forty international investors in New York. Dad and I met from time to time on a casual basis, and at the end of lunch at his favorite Indian restaurant, he brought up Arun. "I didn't know you were so interested in muscle."

His comment surprised me. Arun had been adept at martial arts in his youth and still carried himself with the confidence of a fighter, but did Dad only see him as a chiseled body? Typical for him to be out of touch with reality.

"Maybe you don't know me very well."

SINCE I'D MOVED out of Mom's apartment, I visited her twice a week. She had recovered from her initial outburst and stayed in touch with me throughout the summer in Paris. As Arun had predicted, she refused to pay for her prayers—but he was partly to blame. When he asked her for payment, he quoted eleven-thousand dollars rather than the agreed seven, on the basis that he didn't control the process and her prayers had taken longer than expected. I stayed out of their argument. If he could sense she might not pay, he shouldn't have offered to help her, and to be fair, the significant price increase didn't help. He saw himself as the unfortunate victim in our crossfire, but he had been the one to act rashly.

Mom was the most important person in my life, other than Saby, and despite our differences over Arun, our closeness was unaffected. She was still my anchor, and we returned to the things we enjoyed: conversations, walks, and meals at home with Saby and me at our usual places around the kitchen table.

One Sunday while I was visiting her, Dad showed up unannounced. Since their divorce seven years earlier, their relationship was cordial, but Mom refused to socialize with his wife Lena, and we rarely saw Dad as a family anymore. His presence in Mom's open-plan living room that day was one of those rare occasions. He plopped down on the couch, and we started to chat over cups of coffee. At first it seemed like a normal social call, then out of the blue, Dad pulled himself up to the edge of his seat and faced me square on. His face was puffed out and red. "When are you going to leave him?"

His sudden direct question and the hard edge in his voice caught me off-guard, but I fought to stay composed. "What do you mean? I'm not."

His chest expanded, and he looked like he was going to explode. "You stupid, stupid girl. You know what he is!"

The ferocity of his accusation, so at odds with his usual muted comportment, knocked the wind out of me. A knot of fear rose from my belly to my throat. What was he saying? Did he think Arun was a criminal? Shaken, I stood up and rushed out of the apartment.

Back at home, I collapsed on the bed and sobbed into the pillow, my brain swelling with pain and confusion. I couldn't contact Arun until morning because of the time difference. The hours ahead pressed me into engulfing aloneness.

Then Mom phoned. In a role reversal with Dad, she spoke

in calm, soothing tones. Dad had been upset, that's all; he hadn't meant to lash out. Her call quieted my anguish, and I was able to sleep that night.

Just before waking, I heard Babaji's voice in a dream. "I'm having a party, and you're the guest of honor. But it's up to you if you want to attend or not."

His clear benign presence eased my mind. Of course, I would be there; nothing could keep me from my destiny.

11

SPIRIT INTERVENTION

After a separation of four months, I returned to India at the start of 1996. In the taxi from Delhi to Rishikesh, I picked up an unusual scent. A cloying sweetness surrounded Arun even when the windows were open. I tried to think what it might be until it came to me. "Are you smoking marijuana?"

He answered as if it was evident. "Yes, didn't I tell you?"

My belly tightened with worry. I hadn't smoked or experienced any other drugs, and assumed Arun was the same. "No."

A gentle breeze wafted into the car as we crossed miles of harvested fields. His warm hand covered mine on the seat between us. "I use it for my practices."

Sitting in silence, I glanced at him from time to time. He looked calm, and by the time we reached the mountain house, the grip of fear had loosened.

I settled into our love nest and the quiet rhythm of life surrounded by nature, the place where I had discovered my spiritual path and felt at peace. But Arun continued to test my resolve about spending my life with him.

"You're still young, Jo. You might change your mind."

"I won't."

"What about children?" He peered into my face. "You know I can't have children."

He had told me about his vasectomy in the late sixties, presumably after the dead Arun had already had five children. It was one of those wonderful facts about him, like his circumcision. He'd told me Hindu men didn't get circumcised, only Muslims. "I had it done as soon as I got his body," he told me with pride.

When he spoke about children, he fixed me intently. "There is no force in the universe more powerful than a woman who wants a child. Nothing can stand in her way."

I shook my head. "I don't want children."

"You say this now, and I accept it, but if you change your mind someday, you must tell me."

The desire for children had arisen for a fleeting period in my early days at Harvard when I caught sight of women pushing baby carriages. I imagined their bliss. Perhaps it was a form of escape from the pressure of my new studies. Perhaps I longed for home or a different path, but the feeling passed as quickly as it arose. I became engrossed in my studies and the world of TM, and found my purpose. I didn't need children when the world needed me, and I would devote myself to making it better. Now with my future and spiritual mission taking shape with Arun, I had moved even further from the stable existence of motherhood.

He spoke daily of the other side—a place as real for him as the material world was for others. The elders who lived there were not only his guides but his closest companions. One day, with a somber expression, he made a confession. "I killed an elder once. I didn't mean to, but it happened. They are still punishing me for it."

I couldn't grasp the full meaning of his words. Weren't the elders already dead? Was their punishment the reason for his arrest in California? There was so much about him I still didn't understand, but someday I would.

He reassured me with a gentle smile. "I can't wait for you to remember everything you used to know."

In his hope was the promise of my spiritual development. I wasn't in a rush to get there—it would be unsettling to remember my past lives before I was ready—but his belief in me buoyed me up and kept me going.

We had few contacts with the external world, apart from a handful of families who lived on the adjoining land. They had low-paid jobs at the local English school, and though the children would grow up to speak English, the parents didn't. One of them was a striking young widow. Alone with two young children, she had an even harder time making ends meet, and Arun took a benevolent interest in her. He had dismissed his servant Bahadur and did the cooking himself, but his dishes were too spicy for me. When the widow occasionally brought us food she had made, it was a relief. He mentioned taking her to the dentist to have a broken front tooth capped, an expense she couldn't have afforded, and I was struck by his thoughtfulness and generosity.

With Arun's encouragement and Dad's support, I applied for the MBA program at INSEAD in Fontainebleau, France. It wasn't a choice I would have considered for myself, but Dad had offered to pay for my studies and give me a job when I graduated. I had also spoken to a lawyer about a legal career, which I thought might suit me, but he had also pushed me toward the MBA, which would give me the opportunity to work in any state. I spent a month in Rishikesh, then needed to return to work and prepare for the GMAT entrance exam.

ON A SUNDAY IN MARCH, I went to visit Mom and found her slumped in bed at midday. I sensed immediately something was wrong. She tightened her pink crocheted shawl around her shoulders and asked me to sit.

"Mom, what is it?"

"Your father's been arrested."

"What? What happened?"

She sighed. "Elie just phoned. He's in a jail in Georgia. That's all I know."

They had traveled to the Caspian Sea together for negotiations on the gas pipeline project.

"What can we do?" I asked.

"Elie's in touch with the American Embassy. He'll call when he has news."

It wasn't the first time Dad had been caught up in political turmoil. During his campaign for the Lebanese presidency in the late eighties, he had been kidnapped, and Mom had intervened to secure his release. He managed to leave the country, but the government placed an Interpol warrant for his arrest. He contended that the charges were fabricated to seize his assets and end his campaign; that any law-abiding government would see through the political motivations behind them.

I was sixteen when it happened, and Mom made furtive trips to sell their apartment in Paris and help negotiate Dad's release. Each time, she said she was going to California. I couldn't understand why she felt the need to lie when it was obvious she was going to Paris. But it was a traumatic time for all of us, and I didn't question her. As soon as Dad was released, she initiated divorce proceedings: he had pushed things too far.

When he finally returned to New York, he seemed humbled yet determined to recover his wealth and status. The Interpol warrant hadn't been exercised or stopped him from traveling. The news of his arrest in Georgia was at once shocking and familiar.

I left Mom's room to think for a moment. So little about Dad made sense it was difficult to interpret the situation. Was his arrest a case of political showmanship, or was it a more serious situation? Would he suffer in a Georgian jail?

Mom had been traumatized by her experiences with him and the chaos that trailed him. The situation required exceptional help. I returned to her and asked whether she wanted me to speak with Arun. She gazed out to the wall of windows. "If you want."

I called him immediately, and after listening intently to my words, he spoke in a grave voice. "Do you want me to save your father?"

His tone suggested the worst. In a flash, I saw Dad dying and what would follow: my work with him would stop; I wouldn't pursue the MBA; I would resume my life with Mom and Saby and end my relationship with Arun. Somehow Dad and Arun—their ambitions for me—were linked. Without Dad, the fabric of my life with Arun would unravel.

I answered, "Yes."

"That's all I need to know."

Less than a year after Mom had refused to pay for her prayers, he asked her for six thousand dollars to save Dad's life. A small price to pay.

When Dad and Elie returned from Georgia a few days later, neither one said much about what happened there. Elie smiled when we met at the office and only mentioned his pain from a broken rib. Dad offered no clues. His only message was to have returned unscathed. Arun, on the other hand, spoke of accompanying Dad in spirit form throughout his imprisonment. "I was with him the whole time. If you ask him, he will tell you."

I wouldn't. Even if Dad had sensed him, he wouldn't acknowledge a spiritual presence.

When he and I sat together at his apartment, he shocked me by saying, "I could have introduced you to an oil man. You could get married and make lots of money."

How could he even make such a suggestion? I wouldn't be

a pawn in one of his deals. If I had expected more from Dad, I would have been appalled; instead, I felt a surge of relief. With Arun I could build a different life away from material pursuits.

By April, while I waited for an answer from INSEAD and the work with Elie had reached an impasse, I returned to visit Arun in Rishikesh. It would be my last opportunity in a while if I was admitted to the MBA. It was the start of the summer months in northern India, and waves of heat beat down relentlessly on the house from mid-morning till late into the evening. Daily power cuts in the afternoon coincided with the hottest period of the day; fans hung still while perspiration dripped down my face and back. My head was stuffed with cotton balls, and the only relief was to lie on the cool surface of the cement floor.

The year before I had been there on my birthday and Arun had hardly remembered it, so I had no expectations this year, but he made a point of celebrating. He organized a party with Surat and Usha and ordered a cake from the one bakery in town. Before our guests arrived, he stood in the kitchen door-jamb and made an announcement. The elders wanted to give me a special boon for my birthday: no matter how old I grew, I wouldn't age physically. Even when I turned forty, I'd look the same as at twenty-four. I hadn't given much thought to hanging on to my youth, but the attention of spiritual luminaries brought me joy.

"You're very special to them. They have seven boons for you. I only have five." He smiled at the wonder of it all.

Arun focused a lot on longevity. He said another name for the elders was "time masters" and posed the following quandary. "Imagine a society where you're a child until you're seventy-five; a young man up to one-hundred and fifty. Where you're not old until you reach three hundred."

Only Babaji had ever lived in such a place. But on my

twenty-fourth birthday, forty sounded ancient, and to look young until then was a pleasant boon indeed.

One afternoon, a few days before my return to New York, I was standing in the entrance room of the house when a wooden crate was delivered. Arun carried it to the kitchen and placed it on the counter. When I asked him what it was, he said he had managed to obtain French wine through a connection at the embassy in Delhi. Alcohol, along with meat, was forbidden in Rishikesh; both were considered unholy, and French wine would have been difficult to obtain in India at that time.

I had never seen Arun drink and assumed he was a teetotaler like me. The arrival of the crate was confounding, but before I could ask any more questions, he pressed his thick hands on the counter and dropped his head. When he raised it, he looked at me with a dazed expression, as if he were seeing me for the first time. Instinctively, I stepped back and dropped my head.

He blinked and said, "Mother Joelle, is that you?" A sheen covered his face.

I nodded, sensing a spirit had entered Arun's body.

"It's good to see you. It's not the same from the other side. I'm Tao. You don't know me, but I know who you are."

Tao opened the crate and lifted out a bottle. "You wanted to know about this. It's for the ritual he did to save your father." He focused on me. "He took the help of forces he should not have. We told him not to do it, but he insisted."

He unscrewed the cork and poured himself a glass. A hint of sourness escaped from the bottle. As he took a first sip, he pursed his lips. "He doesn't like it, but he has no choice."

After taking another swallow, he addressed me with a glint in his eyes. "Tell me. What are the pairs of opposites?"

On the spot I couldn't think, and he rattled off, "Sun and moon. Male and female. Light and dark?"

"Yes, yes."

"Everything you see in the world comes from the pairs of opposites. That's the process he's teaching you."

I listened in wonder at this being who had traveled from the other side, who knew everything about our lives here.

"You're progressing well. Keep learning everything you can from him. Someday you might leave him behind."

I didn't want that time to come.

"How long will he need to drink?"

"For some time."

"What about my MBA?"

"You will go and make us all proud."

"I haven't gotten in yet."

"You will." He smiled as if all he had ever wanted to do was stand in this kitchen with me and look out at the world.

Then without warning, Arun's head dropped, and Tao was gone. His eyes took on a wariness absent only moments before. "You met Tao?"

It was hard to believe, but I had. "Are they around us all the time?"

He picked up on my discomfort. "No. They're busy with work on the other side."

After that first meeting, I felt I had been allowed into Arun's secret reality: the hidden world to which he traveled when he slept, the place that marijuana helped him reach. I had felt intimidated in Tao's presence, but the steady tone of his voice was comforting. Different from Arun. Tao was filled with light and reason.

Soon after, we took a taxi to Delhi in the grey haze of dawn, and as I looked out at the hills and the river, tears streamed down my face. It was the first time I left a place crying.

. . .

BACK IN NEW YORK, Dad asked me to leave his apartment as he needed it for visitors, and I reluctantly moved in with Mom. I was apprehensive about living with her again after our disagreement about Arun a year earlier, but she welcomed me back with open arms. She had a lot of work to do at home and spent hours drafting psychological reports, but she made a particular effort to be present and pay attention to me. When Arun went up to his cave in Gangotri, I lost touch with him for a few days and confessed my panic to Mom. What if he never returned and I didn't see him again? She comforted me and said she was sure he would be back. Her calm voice assuaged my anguish.

We went on a short vacation together over the fourth of July to an island off the coast of South Carolina, which I had selected but neither of us knew. The humidity was overpowering, and by late morning, it only took a few steps outside for steam to cover my glasses.

We were relaxing in our respective bedrooms in the air-conditioned bungalow one afternoon when I heard a screeching shout. I ran to see what happened and found Mom lying on her bed, gripping her shoulders. "There." She pointed to the television screen across from her. "There was a dark shadow."

I looked but couldn't see anything.

"It's gone now," she said.

I told Arun about the incident, and he said, "Sometimes the elders get caught in television rays."

When he asked Mom for payment for saving Dad, she refused; denied ever agreeing to it. Once again, he felt cheated, but Mom and I were getting along so well that I wanted to close the matter quickly and told him I would pay. I had started rebuilding my savings from a year of working with Dad.

"That's not the point. She agreed to it. She should honor her side."

"Well, what can we do now?"

"Nothing. It was my stupidity to trust her. The elders warned me not to do it."

"What if you hadn't?"

"He wasn't supposed to survive. I did it for you."

PART II

MAKING A LIVING

12

TOGETHER

In late August, two weeks before the start of classes at INSEAD, I still didn't have an offer of admission. Arun and I were staying at the worn-out studio Dad kept for guests in Paris. Meeting in France had been Arun's idea: he was sure I would get in. When my confidence flagged, he repeated one of his favorite phrases, "It's not over till it's over."

Then, as if by magic, I received a message from the university: another student had fallen ill, did I want to join? I couldn't believe my sudden good fortune, and Arun credited the elders for the turn of events. As long as we remained true to them through our practice, they would work things out for us from the other side. I had doubted the outcome, but he had turned out to be right.

With my access to Dad's business checkbook and signatory power, I made out a check for the deposit to register my place. When I informed Dad, he seemed slightly taken aback but said nothing more. He had promised to pay for my studies, and I didn't want to give him the chance to change his mind and risk losing the opportunity.

Arun and I had spoken of getting married in France, and he

had bought our gold wedding bands in India. When I went to campus for the first time, I wore it and informed the administrators I would be attending with my husband. We would marry soon, and I was eager to present our relationship as solid and final.

There was one remaining ad on campus for student accommodation: a penthouse in the town of Fontainebleau about a twenty-minute walk away. It was in a small building up five flights of stairs, and after a quick look around, we signed the lease immediately.

A week later, I sat in a darkened amphitheater filled with hundreds of students. Professors stood at the central podium and expounded their theories of economics, accounting, and finance while pointing at projected slides. At twenty-four, I was younger than most of my classmates and far less experienced. At question time, they were so eager: formulating eloquent, coherent responses to business problems I hadn't even considered. For the first time, I felt out of place in an academic setting. I listened and fidgeted in my seat while my mind traveled to Arun at home.

Shortly after we arrived, he announced that he would audit my classes so we could learn at the same time; but once the classes were underway, he gave up on the idea. He wanted me to find my own place and had other concerns. He found French wine and drank it in large quantities. The arrival of the crate in Rishikesh had coincided with the appearance of Tao. I had been taken by his visit and hadn't considered what Arun meant by a ritual offering to the dark side to save Dad's life. I expected him to drink a glass or two, but an entire bottle became his usual dose. And when he discovered a local forty-proof liqueur, allegedly made by monks, he added it to his daily fare. Overnight the man I had known as a teetotaler wallowed in the effects of alcohol.

I would return from a day of struggling with my new

studies to find him sitting on the couch, legs stretched out and ankles crossed over the coffee table, watching the *Jerry Springer* show, chuckling at the contestants' extreme behavior. An empty glass lay at his side. When I asked why he was watching such an inane program, he responded, "It's nothing. Just a bit of fun."

If he had more of the liqueur that day, he tottered to the kitchen, eyes glassy and unfocused. His new habit filled me with anguish; but when I expressed it, he only stared with unrecognizable blankness. If I insisted too much, his eyes hardened, and his mouth tightened. How did a yogi who communed with the elders put himself in such a state? All I could do was wait for the hours to pass. The inexplicable change in Arun, two years after we met, was like finding out the earth is flat.

He spoke of the dark forces he was fighting off, but said if they ever succeeded in taking over his body, I should call his guardian spirits for help. Sitting on the floor of the small room at the back of the apartment where I had set up our computer, he taught me their names: Udo and Mado. They were spirits who had never had a body and had been created by the elders for a single purpose: protecting or taking life. If a dark force ever managed to take over his body, it would demand meat, and I should call out to Udo, then leave the apartment immediately.

"Practice saying his name," he said.

I dragged the first syllable. "Oodo."

"No, not like that. U-do."

I repeated the two short syllables.

"That's better."

I was alarmed at the thought of an evil spirit entering Arun's body. Would I recognize the signs? Would I remember the correct pronunciation of Udo's name? I hoped it would never come to that.

In the meantime, I did my best to accept his drinking, but his state of mind soon affected our intimacy. From a man who had been tender in sexual relations, he became an unfeeling mechanical partner. Since he didn't tolerate any discussion about his drinking, I lay still and waited for the moment to pass. But he didn't take well to my indifference and asked what the matter was.

"Nothing, I'm just tired."

"It's not nothing."

My heart thumped in the silence of the dark room.

"You're always tired."

I forced an exhale. "It's the studies. They're taking a lot out of me."

He sounded determined. "It's something else. Tell me what it is."

My belly knotted up.

"You're not attracted to me anymore."

"It's not that."

"Then?"

I took a moment to compose my thoughts. "You don't feel like yourself when you've been drinking."

"Nothing has changed. Why do you say that?"

"I just feel it."

"You know why I'm drinking." He made it sound as if I was knocking him down when he was already low.

The sound of the clock ticking felt oppressive. "How long will it last?"

"Some time."

I pushed myself up and sat by his side. "But it will end someday, right?"

He looked at me through the darkness. "Someday, yes."

His answer was too vague. I needed a timeframe: six months, a year—anything to help me face the days ahead.

. . .

WE WENT to the city hall in Fontainebleau to find out the administrative requirements for marriage, and returned with a date for the civil ceremony at the end of October and a list of required paperwork. We also had to present the results of HIV tests, and I was relieved to find out we were both negative. Arun had told me of his many lovers and a period of sexual excess from which he had reformed. It took several weeks to obtain birth certificates and other necessary documents from our respective embassies, but we finally gathered everything needed before the ceremony.

One afternoon, while I sat at the dining table and sunlight poured through the skylights into the open space living room, Arun bent on one knee and peered up at me with his deer eyes. He clasped the *mangalsutra,* a thin gold chain with a filigreed heart pendant, around my neck. While he was still in India, I had researched the Hindu symbol of marriage and asked him to bring me one.

Then he said, more formally than I expected, "Will you marry me?"

"Yes."

There was no doubt in my mind. Since I had gone to his hotel room in Delhi and told him I loved him, and he revealed I had been his wife, I had no other wish. Whatever trouble we were facing now, we would overcome it. And I wasn't going to ask Mom or Dad for permission. I was old enough to marry, mature enough to know who I loved. By the time I reached puberty, I had made up my mind and told them both my view in a rare family moment in Mom's living room. "Love is finding the whole world in someone else and needing to look no more." Dad had smiled at my youthful idealism, but it was my challenge to them. And though I had dated other men, I had been saving myself for my future husband: the one love that would last forever.

Mom and Dad had their secrets—hidden extramarital

affairs—without considering Saby and me. They hadn't been true to each other and never explained why, or what they really did want. But my path was different: I had excelled in high school, graduated from a top university, and now started advanced studies. I could decide by myself and enter into a life-long bond with Arun.

One morning shortly after our marriage, I found him sitting at the dining table sobbing into his hands. I had never seen him cry before and rushed to his side. He wiped his eyes and looked up at me. "I saw my parents for the first time last night. They are giants, huge, not from this world." He looked like a lost child who had found home. Then he smiled. "My mother told me to treat you with respect. Not like the men down here." He took me in his arms and held me. This was the Arun I knew—deep, spiritual, loving—the one he would become again after the drinking ritual was over.

WHILE I FOCUSED on my classes, he had taken on domestic responsibilities: cooked our meals, cleaned the apartment, and gave me a massage once a week. I meditated every day before going to campus after a much-reduced physical yoga practice: one prolonged standing forward bend. Arun called it the "queen of all postures" and believed holding the pose for twenty minutes or more extended life. I could never achieve that feat: a few minutes in, my head would buzz with pressure, and I kneeled to the floor.

The autumn cold had set in, and I returned from classes one evening with the usual weariness of the day. The apartment was dark, and Arun sat on the couch in a drink-fueled daze. I was used to his long afternoon travels when he lay down to nap and sent his spirit to work. I flicked on the lights and went into the kitchen. A bottle of liqueur sat empty on the counter, dark purple dregs pooled at the bottom. I brought it out to the living room and held it up to him. "This bottle is empty."

He staggered up, stared at the bottle, and narrowed his eyes in a silent frown.

"Didn't you just buy it yesterday?"

"Are you checking?" He walked past me to the kitchen.

"Well, you seem drunk."

He forced his eyes open. "I'm not drunk."

The room was bathed in an orange glow, and I went to sit at the dining table. "It's too much. You're going to hurt yourself."

He turned to me. "Is there something you want to tell me?"

I shook my head. "I'm worried, that's all."

His voice gained strength. "Please. I want to know. You know why I'm doing this." The sudden harshness of his tone sucked the air from the room. I looked down in silence.

He stood by the table. "I sit here all day. Wait for you. Then you come home, and this is all you have to say to me."

My heart tightened, and I forced in a breath. "I'm sorry. It's just . . ." Why had I accused him? If only I could un-see the bottle and un-speak my words.

He stepped away toward the kitchen. "This isn't a life."

"Wait. I'm sorry. I didn't mean to say anything bad."

Suddenly wide awake, he turned to me, like a man possessed.

"This isn't going to work."

"What?"

"You heard me. This isn't going to work. I want out."

My heart squeezed in my chest. This shouldn't be happening.

"What are you talking about? We just got married."

His presence, so close yet so punishing, was suffocating.

He looked away and spoke with the slow deliberateness of an actor delivering a speech.

"I can see it now. You don't love me. I don't know how I missed it before."

"Don't say that! I love you."

He returned to face me, but I had lost him. "No, you don't. You thought you did. You would never accuse me like that if you loved me."

The room felt like a trap. "I didn't accuse you."

He walked to the master bedroom at the back, returned with his passport, and placed it on the dining table. "I'll leave tomorrow." He removed his wedding ring and lay it on the passport. "I won't need this anymore."

"Arun-ji, don't say this!" I addressed him with the honorific -ji, which I sometimes used lovingly.

He went to sit on the couch and remained silent.

I trailed behind him and knelt by his side. "I'm sorry if I said something wrong. I didn't realize you would drink hard alcohol."

"Leave me alone."

Sobs erupted from deep within me. "I can't leave you alone, Arun-ji. I love you. I don't want to be without you."

"Get up. I don't want to see you."

His words felt like a punch to my belly. I returned to the dining table and held my head in my hands. The tightness in my chest was unbearable. A well of darkness surrounded me. How had we come to this point? I wished I could be transported anywhere else.

When I finally left the room and went to bed, I lay in torment, drowning in thoughts of loss. The loss of his trust. The reversal of his love and affection so soon after his mother's instruction to treat me well. The abandonment of the MBA, which I wouldn't complete without him. Worst of all, a return to the life I had known before, without his guidance and link to the other side. That sense of being adrift before we met—I would do almost anything not to return there.

After what felt like hours, I fell into a fitful sleep.

The next morning, I walked tentatively into the living room. He was sitting quietly in the same place where I had left him, but his face was more open. I renewed the same pleas in a calmer tone, and he relented. Later he put his passport away. We had narrowly escaped separation, and I had survived a dark night, but I was on guard.

One day Arun mentioned Mom's parents. They had died in my early childhood, before Saby's birth, and their loss had left Mom devastated. He said I wouldn't be with him if they were still alive. As if the family rupture had pulled us apart and left me vulnerable. I didn't agree: I couldn't imagine a life in which I was better off without him.

13

LIFELINE

I got to know my classmates and introduced them to Arun. The wives accompanying the many male students took a liking to him, and he started a free yoga class on campus. As I had already seen in India, he had a polarizing effect on men and was quick to point out the Indian engineer who didn't like him. It didn't bother me. Not everyone needed to like him; and though I was proud of my yogi husband, we weren't the typical couple.

Before the Christmas break, I called Dad to ask for the balance of the university fees, which were due in the new year.

His answer was swift. "I don't have it."

"What do you mean you don't have it?"

"I don't have the money right now."

"But you promised to pay for my MBA."

"Things happen, Jo."

"What am I supposed to do now?"

"Do what everyone else does. Apply for a loan."

I twirled the telephone cord in my hand. "There isn't much time. What if I don't get a loan?"

"Then stop for some time. It's not the end of the world. You can go back and finish later."

I couldn't believe it: he was casually reneging on his promise. I knew him to be unreliable, but his brusque tone and lack of concern churned my belly. After being adamant about my completing an MBA, he was acting like it didn't matter. And how could he be flush with money one day and empty the next? Even if I didn't believe him, there was nothing I could do about it. I had completed almost half the coursework and wouldn't stop now.

Arun and I separated over the break. He went to India to apply for a long-term visa, now as the spouse of a student in France, and I returned to New York. Before leaving, he bought a heap of secondhand fur-lined leather jackets from the outdoor market and piled them on the couch. I marveled at the quantity and at his excitement. He wanted to sell them or give them away in Rishikesh.

Back home, I asked Mom if she would let me include her tax returns in my student loan application; the financial information could help me qualify for a more favorable interest rate, but I doubted she would openly share them with me. Mom and Dad were both secretive about their finances. She blamed him for stopping all payments to her after his kidnapping and eventual release, and he accused her of taking everything he had. The upshot was I didn't know the reality of their financial situations. As expected, Mom brushed off my question, and I completed the application on my own. When the loan was approved, I paid the remaining course fees and had sufficient funds for us to live in Fontainebleau for the rest of the academic year.

The first two academic terms before Christmas had been fraught with tension at home, and I had difficulty concentrating on my studies. But by the third term exams, Arun was away in India, and my mind focused freely. We had moved beyond the foundation courses of accounting, finance, and economics, and I earned a top mark in business strategy. In the final two terms, we had more choice, and I focused on entrepreneurship. Ever since I learned TM at the age of eighteen, I wanted to teach the healing power of meditation. Arun and I would start a well-being business, and I wrote a business plan to open a resort in the countryside outside Paris. Our shared mission would bring back his drive, purpose, and light.

Despite my dream, as the year came to an end, I needed to find a job. Dad wasn't ready to hire me into his business, and I would need a corporate sponsor to be able to stay in Europe. I decided that if I had to work for a company—a prospect I wasn't especially looking forward to—it would be in the high tech industry, which in the late nineties was on the brink of changing society. I didn't know how to go about approaching companies on my own, so I focused on the one that came to recruit on campus: a Canadian telecommunications supplier called Nortel. Not exactly high tech, but close enough; and at least it wasn't consumer goods, which I couldn't bring myself to consider.

On the day of the interview, I wore a new pinstriped suit and stood in line behind one of my classmates, a Spanish man who knew and respected Arun. He turned back to look at me and flicked a piece of lint from my shoulder. I smiled and thanked him. I needed to make my best impression. When he completed his own interview, he paused before walking on and whispered the most challenging question in my ear. I gathered my thoughts over the next minute and had an answer ready when they asked.

June was our final month in Fontainebleau, and though the student loan had seemed more than sufficient to cover our expenses, our bank account was already close to depleted. I hadn't kept a budget. It didn't seem necessary just to pay rent, utilities, and food. Arun did all the shopping, and no single purchase stood out, but now I had to monitor the account to make sure we wouldn't go into overdraft.

We were walking back from campus one day when he paused in front of the display of a computer store on our street, then went in without a word. I followed him, and he showed me a reactive joystick. It was nine-hundred francs (a hundred euros), and he wanted to buy it. I refused. Not only was it too expensive, but he wasn't a serious gamer.

He ignored me and asked a salesperson to get him one.

"We can't afford it."

When the salesperson returned with the box, Arun repeated, "I want it." He took it to the counter and paid for it from our joint bank account.

With a large shopping bag in his hand, he stopped dead on the pavement outside, his eyes hard and cold. "Don't you ever stand up to me like that in public again."

I smarted from the reprimand, and silently absorbed the sickening realization that we would run out of money before I had found a job.

WITH ARUN'S reputation on campus as a yogi and therapist, an Israeli student came to him with back pain. After a few massages his back was healed, and he raved about Arun's abilities. He would have taken his advanced yoga course if he could afford it. When his mother came to Fontainebleau, Arun invited them home for a meal, and she presented him with a small box with two tiny diamonds. After they left, I expected him to give them to me, but he placed the box with his belongings. He wanted to have them mounted into studs for himself on his next trip to India.

When I eventually told Mom about our marriage, apart from surprising me with her tender tone, she kept quiet. She didn't see Arun the way I did; I doubted she ever would.

Arun bolstered my confidence. He stood in the galley kitchen and looked into my eyes. "Jo, you're my soldier, you know that. You're standing up against the whole world for me." I was proud to stand up for him. My family might reel, but when tested, I would overcome.

They all came for my graduation: not only Mom, Saby, and Dad, but also my aunt Mireille, who lived in Lebanon, and my paternal grandmother from Egypt. Mom took me shopping in Paris and bought me a baby-blue linen dress with a deep V-neck and buttons down the middle. Though the dress was long, it was a change from the plain modest attire I had adopted since meeting Arun. On graduation day one of my classmates commented, "You look beautiful." He had befriended Arun and me at the beginning of the course, but we had been out of touch for a while. I avoided his gaze.

I told my Spanish classmate about my follow-up interview with Nortel in Paris. He was an engineer, and I assumed he was in the same position. When he said he hadn't been called back, I expressed my dismay.

"Don't worry about it." He held my hand longer than I expected. "Good luck."

On one of our last days in the apartment, Arun leaned into the couch and announced, "Now that you have your diploma don't expect me to work. I'm retired."

He sounded pleased with my achievement, but his comment surprised me. I was twenty-five, but at fifty-eight, he was young for an adept of the secret practice. And as he'd shown with the Israeli student, he had so much to offer the world.

"But you'll still teach yoga, right?"

"If the right student comes. But don't expect me to bring in any money."

"I hope I get the job at Nortel."

"You will, you'll see."

Our belongings had multiplied from the two suitcases with which we had arrived, and once they were all packed—the reactive joystick deep within our clothes—only our wedding gifts remained on the mantel of the empty apartment. The glass decanter and ceramic vase were now the only signs that we had been there. I looked at their delicate forms, the joy they had brought me on our special day. "We forgot to wrap them."

"Leave them."

"I want a memory of our wedding."

"They'll break."

It felt wrong to leave behind our only wedding gifts—especially as they were from our landlord—but rather than press the point, I gave in.

My first year living with Arun had taken its toll. We had had recurring fights and become sexually estranged. He was adamant that something was wrong, that I no longer loved him, and every few weeks, his mood spilled into outpourings of rage. On my part, I couldn't get past his glassy eyes and regain my unselfconscious approach to intimacy. And I knew better than to tell him the truth.

Back in Paris after my graduation, we had run out of money, but after a second round of interviews, Nortel offered me a job. I would start in September. I borrowed two thousand dollars from Mom and promised to pay her back from my first salary. Arun and I would return to our respective countries over the summer and apply for residency visas.

A few days before we separated, he took me in his arms and looked at me with tenderness. He forgave me for my reticence, and I turned to kiss him. We found each other again, and the worst seemed to be over.

In the comfort of Mom's house, I found the peace and stability I lacked in my own space. She wanted me to stay and leave Arun, but I wouldn't. I had a lifeline and a plan.

14

GLASS PRISON

I returned to Paris in September, a few days ahead of Arun, and moved into Dad's studio, which he had agreed to lend us for a while. Whatever had caused Dad's sudden and momentary fury about Arun had dissipated, and he had returned to being a quiet onlooker in my life. Two different dark-patterned wallpapers, unchanged since the seventies, covered the walls and peeled at the seams. The thin carpet creased and lifted from the floor. I stayed there for a day, then felt the walls closing in on me, the absence of light clouding my mind. I left and went to stay in a small guest room at Dad's until Arun returned.

My new office was in the La Défense business district just outside Paris, and from the sealed tower, I contemplated the sunrays reflecting from adjacent skyscrapers. I sat alone in a large space with four desks until my permanent place, which I would share with a colleague, became available. I had just missorted the columns in the Excel spreadsheet with names and salaries. My mind blurred, and I let it settle before starting the work all over again. I knew little of the software when I joined the company, but now my role in sales commissions depended on it.

My boss, Richard, headed the sales operations department for one of the company's divisions. About ten years older than me and an accountant by training, he was lightyears ahead in business experience. He was friendly but somewhat aloof, and offered little guidance about the job other than suggesting I call colleagues and find out what the issues were.

I made it through the day by challenging myself to limit the number of times my eyes drifted to the clock. Despite my sedentary work and Richard's absence of pressure, I left the office weighed by exhaustion. When we met in the evenings, Arun had spent his day walking around town and watching television. We inhabited two different worlds, and mine felt like a glass prison.

Since I had started the job toward the end of September, my salary would only be paid at the end of October. I not only wanted to return Mom's loan, but also needed money for living expenses. I went to the Human Resources office and asked if I could receive an advance at the end of the month. To my relief, the advisor granted my request. We wouldn't have made it another five weeks without it.

Dad's studio was only a short walk from where he lived with Lena, and she invited us to lunch on a Saturday. Despite its huge footprint, their apartment only had a few large rooms. Lunch was served at one end of the massive living room, on the antique mahogany desk that used to be Dad's command center in my childhood, back when two ivory elephant tusks stood by the back wall and framed the desk. They had been sold long ago, and the desk became a dining table.

Dad asked me about my job, and when I explained about my responsibility for sales commissions and bonuses, he smirked. "So, you're a bean counter like Edouard?"

Edouard was his father, who had built his own automobile parts business from scratch after leaving Lebanon for Egypt before World War II. He had managed it well and converted his profits into lucrative property investments, leaving Dad with a significant fortune when he died. But Dad didn't value his cautious and methodical approach to business and life. If it didn't involve one massive deal that would change the world, he wasn't interested.

He left after lunch, and Lena offered us Turkish coffee in the sitting area on the opposite side of the room. She had invested in two new couches, but the same shiny black block table from the seventies was still there. When Arun excused himself for a moment, she said to me, "He doesn't love you. He doesn't look at you when you're together."

Despite the absence of malice, her words and lack of sensitivity shocked me. No one had addressed me so directly before about Arun's feelings. But she was wrong. What did she know about love? She had married Dad.

A few weeks later, they hosted a Halloween party and didn't invite us. Arun was offended by the oversight and asked me to confront Dad. I didn't see the need for it, but Arun insisted. When I called Dad and asked why we had been excluded, he said, "We don't want to socialize with you. Your relationship is not biologically normal."

Lena was eighteen years younger; when did a relationship become "biologically normal"?

Another time when Dad and I were alone at his apartment, he commented that, as a mixed-race couple, Arun and I wouldn't be approved for a bank loan. His bigotry shocked me. Surely, he didn't believe what he was saying. When the conversation ended, as he was leaving the room, he turned to me at the last minute. "You took him from me. He and I would have been best friends if it weren't for you."

At first I was stunned—was he jealous of my relationship with Arun? But then I felt vindicated in my choice of partner. I left the apartment, shutting the heavy door behind me, and scampered down the four flights of the broad staircase. The same smell of wood polish wafted up to my nostrils as if no time had passed since my childhood visits.

After we moved into his studio, Dad asked to borrow two thousand euros, and though money was tight after the lean summer months, I felt obligated to lend him the money since we weren't paying rent.

One evening when I got back from work, Arun was nowhere to be found. It was late for him to still be out, and I phoned his mobile, the new device he had insisted on buying during our last days in Fontainebleau. Despite my initial resistance, when he chose the best Nokia model, I bought a simpler one, and now I couldn't imagine not having it. He didn't answer, and I tried again fifteen minutes later. Still nothing. On my third attempt, the call went right to voicemail. It was close to seven, and my mind spiraled into a panic. Where could he be? Had something happened to him? Was he in an accident? I tried to distract myself with tasks around the house, but doom-filled thoughts kept intruding.

He walked in just after seven, and I rushed to greet him. "Where have you been? I've been worried sick."

His brow creased, and he met my emotion with a steely tone. "Why are you talking to me like this? Am I a dog that should wait by the door for you to come home?"

"No, of course not." Swept up by my own anxiety, I had spoken without thinking. I now regretted it.

He had been to his marijuana dealer and was on the metro when I called. No matter how I phrased my apology, his stance didn't soften. Once more, I had been tried and found guilty.

He had met the dealer through a common contact shortly after we arrived in Paris. She lived on the other side of the city, and he visited her regularly for a supply of his favorite herb. He smoked on the balcony, exhaling into the sky, and though I worried about neighbors picking up the scent, marijuana provided a welcome break from his raging alcohol-fueled outbursts. Smoking restored the calm yogi I had known and loved, and I hoped someday it would completely replace drinking.

As Christmas was coming up, I spoke to him about visiting Mom and Saby.

"You're married now. You shouldn't leave your husband for Christmas."

It was the first time he had expressed any disapproval about my travels home, but maybe he felt more vulnerable now, and though I would have preferred to go to New York, I was touched by his sentiment and acquiesced.

When I told Mom, she said, "But he doesn't celebrate Christmas."

"It doesn't matter. He's my husband, and I shouldn't leave him over the holidays."

If no one was going to care about Arun, then I would.

By the start of the new year, I was ready to look for our own place, and told Dad we would leave his studio as long as he repaid my loan. Eager to have his place back, he returned my money, and I called on the property-finding service the company had offered in my joining package. We rented a one-bedroom apartment on a quiet tree-lined street near the Bois de Boulogne and bought a bed, a small couch, and a television. Dad gave us a table and chairs he didn't need.

Over the winter we tried judo classes at a municipal gym—a reminiscence of Arun's martial arts past. It wasn't his first time since we moved to France; he had taken a class in Fontainebleau but found it too strenuous and never returned. After I got used to the way the instructor controlled the class, I enjoyed the focus and effort of the practice, but Arun once again didn't take to it, and we dropped the idea. Instead, we bought four judo mats of our own, placed them across the living room, and used them for our meditation and stretches.

In May, Richard called me into his office. His desk took up most of the room, and I sat across from him. He swiveled toward me, crossed his arms on the table, and leaned in. "When you first joined us, you were so quiet, I wasn't sure if you would fit in." He paused for a moment and looked at me. "But you've really come out of your shell. You've done some great work with the commission payments."

"Thank you." All I had done was bring consistency where there had been disorder, but I could see how the new process would appeal to him.

Then he explained that Nortel had just acquired a data networking company to complement its telecommunications offering. The new company was overrun with sales payment issues, and he wanted me to lead the team of commissions analysts. One was in the UK, and two were in Valbonne. As part of the new job, I would need to move to the South of France. He paused, then added, "You would be promoted to manager."

I digested his messages: how I had come across before settling into the job; the contributions I had made; and the offer of relocation and promotion so soon after we had settled into our own place in Paris. I told Richard I would discuss it with my husband and get back to him.

The salary increase would be substantial, and the promotion to manager less than a year after joining the company wasn't something to take lightly. Arun agreed I should accept the offer, and as part of the agreement, I negotiated French lessons for him since we would be in a small town rather than the cosmopolitan capital.

We would need a car to get around, another significant lifestyle change. We went to a Honda dealership with the intention of buying a new small SUV, but when I discovered a used luxury Legend for the same price, we chose it instead. That was one aspect of life I relished with Arun: nothing was fixed; plans and purchases could change on the spot.

I scheduled a meeting with our banking advisor in Fontainebleau to apply for a car loan on the following Saturday morning, but on the day Arun announced nonchalantly that he had an appointment with the drug dealer.

My eyes opened wide. "Today? Cancel it. We need the loan."

My determined tone must have set him off because he glared at me and accused me of jealousy. I had met the dealer only once and had no interest in returning to her empty loft at the top of a walk-up building. But my insistence on the need to co-sign the loan had nothing to do with personal animosity. He finally agreed to join me, but his displeasure festered throughout the day, and on our return from the bank, he sat quietly on the couch while June's long rays filtered through the door windows. I dreaded the conversation he wanted to have.

When he turned to me and asked what was wrong, I said, "Nothing," but he didn't give up so easily.

"What is it, Jo? Tell me."

"Nothing."

His voice remained steady. "There is something. I know it."

I sighed. Since moving in together at INSEAD, something had changed. The peace I had once felt in his presence had ceded to deep unrest. I searched my mind for a reason. Since he started drinking, I had lost my spontaneity with him—as if sex were a performance I was destined to fail. Even worse were the fights that would follow. Along with my innocence, something else had gone: the feeling that our relationship was safe, and somehow everything would turn out all right. I had made a promise on my wedding day to always tell him the truth. Now was the time to make good on it.

I looked into his eyes and said, "I'm not as attracted to you as I used to be."

He nodded slowly, as if my words confirmed what he already knew.

Immediately, I realized my mistake.

In a calm even tone, he said, "I want a divorce."

His words dealt a clean blow to my diaphragm. "Arun, no, don't say that."

"You said it yourself."

"I, I. You pushed me."

His gentle eyes rested on mine. "It's okay. It's better this way. The truth always comes out."

"No, it's not better." My voice rose. "I love you."

"You say this now, and I believe you, but someday, somewhere, you will leave me. And it will be too difficult for me then."

"I won't."

I spoke through sobs, fighting to convince him, but he sat impervious to my pleas. I would have done anything to take back what I said, but it was too late. I couldn't change his mind and later that evening, I retired to the bedroom alone.

The bedside lamp cast a shadow on the walls. I envisioned the impossible path I would tread alone. I didn't even know how to drive, didn't feel up to taking a job in a new place where I knew no one. But it wasn't so much the practical matters that worried me—I could quit my job and return to the US if I had to. I didn't want to separate from Arun. Whatever troubles besieged us in the material world, we were soul mates, reunited across lifetimes. We had already overcome so much to stay together, I wouldn't give up now.

I bolted out of bed and went to find him. He was still sitting in the living room where I had left him, and I crouched by his side. I renewed my impassioned pleas, but he begged me to leave him alone. Finally, he took hold of one of our bamboo exercise poles and pointed it in my direction, inches from my arm. The expression in his eyes didn't match the force of his gesture, but I took the point and returned to bed.

I slept little that night and awoke the next morning under the weight of exhaustion. Arun was already dressed and ready to leave.

I coaxed him again in a quieter tone. "Let me make it up to you."

"You can't." He sounded like he was reasoning with a child.

"I don't want you to leave."

"I'll book my flight today. Please don't try to hold me back."

"How did we come to this?"

He looked at me. "As soon as I leave, you'll forget everything you learned from me. The elders will make sure the knowledge is erased from your mind."

I swallowed. "I won't be part of their family?"

"No. That will end."

A gentle breeze filtered through the open windows. A warm bright Sunday morning would have been the perfect time for a walk in the woods if the situation had been different.

"I'll call my parents."

"You do that."

I called Dad—Mom wouldn't be awake yet in New York—and he was better in a crisis anyway. I told him about Arun's decision and the words that had set him off. It was the first time I was confiding with anyone about our marital troubles.

"You told him that?" Dad responded.

I realized then I had overstepped a line with Arun.

Dad was out of town and said that Lena would be in touch.

I phoned Mom later and told her Arun had requested a divorce. She sounded pressured by the news. She had a full load of patients but would review her schedule and try to fly to Paris on the weekend. When we hung up, I felt like I had imposed my problems on her, and wasn't sure whether she would be able to travel. Maybe she hoped Dad would handle the situation.

Arun said he would make his travel plans on Monday, and the day passed in silence. That night, a female figure appeared in my dream and brought comfort to my fitful mind. I woke up feeling hopeful and told Arun about the dream.

The wind of rage had blown from his face. He contemplated me with calm eyes. "You saw Mother, Babaji's female form. She is the most powerful on the other side."

I sat by him. "I felt her presence. I know she was there."

"You're a very special person if she appeared to you."

A glimmer of light parted the clouds of despair.

"What do you want me to do, Jo? Just tell me, and I'll do it."

I had no doubt in my mind. "I want you to stay."

"Are you sure that's what you want?"

"Yes."

He turned his gaze to the window, then returned to me. "If you want me to, I will."

I had been waiting two days for him to change his mind; it was a hard-won recovery.

"Let me say one thing." He stared at me and raised his large open hands. "If you ever fall in love with another man, you must tell me before anything happens. It will be very painful for me, but if you tell me the truth, I will accept it. But if I ever find out that you went with someone behind my back, I will kill you both." His eyes flinched.

"I won't cheat on you."

"I'm warning you: I won't be able to handle it."

His command seemed both extreme and romantic; his threat of violence a natural consequence of his passion. Did he love me that much?

There was no risk: I didn't want anyone else.

15

SAND THROUGH OPEN FINGERS

By the time Lena got in touch, the rift between Arun and me had mended. She invited us for lunch at their country club and chatted with us more openly than before. It felt like she and Dad had decided to reverse their earlier rejection of our relationship and see us through a rough period as a new couple. Whenever we met up with her, Arun was charming, self-possessed, and engaging, and she welcomed the connection with us.

On her last visit to our home before we moved to the south, Arun had prepared his signature spicy shrimp dish, and she opened up about Dad. She was concerned about his repeated business setbacks. Time and again, he threw himself wholeheartedly into a highly lucrative opportunity, working for years without payment, only for it to crumble at the last minute.

"I'm sad for him, not for me."

Arun listened with attention and responded to her concern. "Someone might have left a jinx there. I might be able to help you, but you will need to follow my instructions exactly. Otherwise his luck will get worse."

She pondered his words and wondered whether a former

employee who had left their apartment unwillingly, when it ceased being an office, might be behind his spell of bad luck. She agreed to Arun's intervention, and he went there the following day. After surveying the place, he confirmed the presence of something untoward, smeared blood on the inside of the main door frame, and instructed Lena to leave the stains untouched for three days. But when Dad returned from a trip early and saw the marks, he was furious with her for succumbing to idle superstition and demanded that she clean the blood immediately.

Arun heard the news and shook his head. "That's what I get for trying to help. His situation will be very bad."

I worried for Dad, though I didn't believe his fate depended entirely on the ritual. Like my distrust for playing the Lotto, something held me back from magical thinking. And I couldn't help but think that Arun had set Lena up for failure. In the same way his efforts on Mom's behalf had backfired.

Then Tao made an appearance. He visited from time to time through Arun's body, but unlike his host, he was unaffected by alcohol. In his calm and comforting manner, he acted as the mediator and spoke of Arun as a hot-headed child. I trusted his wisdom and told him about the confrontation between Dad and Lena over the ritual.

He shook his head. "Your father will never change. He was the same last time also."

I stopped and stared. "You know him?"

He paused for a moment. "Yes, he was my father, too. You were my sister." He smiled gently, "When I came down from the mountains, you took care of me. I owe you a lot."

I was stunned by the revelation of our former closeness. "Where were we?"

I expected him to say China, the land of the Taoist stories.

"Benares. You lived there."

Arun had never mentioned the holy Hindu city nor suggested a visit there.

"You were a rich woman. A widow. Our mother died when we were young. Our father was a fraud back then, too."

Growing up without a mother must have been lonely, as would being a widow. Perhaps that was why Arun had taken pity on our neighbor raising two children on her own: she reminded him of me.

"Arun said terrible things would happen to Dad."

"He will never change. Whatever money comes to him will flow out of his hands like sand from open fingers." He opened his palms and splayed his fingers in the air. "I warned Arun not to interfere, but he wanted to. He cares about you too much."

THE FIRST TIME I received correspondence from the bank addressing me by my married name, it looked odd. I hadn't requested the change, but the bank had assumed, perhaps after the joint car loan, that I shared Arun's surname. I hadn't considered changing my maiden name before, but transitioning from Dad's daughter to Arun's wife was appealing. I would make my bond to him even more explicit and take control of my adult life.

Dad's name came with baggage I would prefer not to carry. Like when one of the few American students at INSEAD, an imposing woman in a tight-fitted skirt and heels, had marched toward me in the cafeteria and said, "Are you related to Roger Tamraz?"

"Yes, he's my father."

She pursed her lips. "I almost lost my job because of him."

She had been working in Washington at the time of Dad's Senate hearings relating to his large donations to the Democratic party. He hadn't been found guilty of wrongdoing, but she made it sound as if I was responsible somehow. I didn't know how to respond to her, and she walked away.

It had been the only incident in the recent past, but who knew when someone else would link us up and expect me to explain what I didn't know? I was a working woman now, soon to be responsible for a team; it was time to adopt my new identity as Arun's wife.

IN VALBONNE, an inland town on the French Riviera, our life changed. After a failed attempt to teach me to drive the Legend, Arun took me to and from the office, a fifteen-minute journey. We lived in a house on a large plot, and I had hoped that the new scenery and glorious sunshine would uplift his mood, but within days, gloom descended upon him. Despite the brand-new building, terracotta floor tiles, and spacious open-plan living area, he said the wooden doors were flimsy and the construction was cheap. Tao drank freely from the bottle of newly discovered Pastis, the local anise liqueur, but after he left, Arun was groggy and worn.

At work, my team was challenging, and the work needed to implement a better payment process took time and effort. At home, Arun's somber state seeped into my mind, and I felt weary and alone. When I didn't respond as he expected in bed, he renewed his pointed interrogations and questioned my affections. I knew better than to respond to his demands for explanations and deflected his harangues while willing the moment to pass. My husband was a paradox: a yogi with deep otherworldly knowledge and an irate man I couldn't please.

One evening, though it looked like Arun, a different being came to pick me up from work. I realized right away something was off: the spirit in his body didn't utter a word—apart from the occasional grunt—and drove at a constant high speed even through sharp winding turns. Although he seemed in control of the vehicle, I clung to the door until we reached the house. Once we were inside, Arun returned. He shook off whatever influence had been inside him moments earlier and looked at me apologetically. "Sorry I couldn't reach you in time."

When Mom and Saby came for a visit, I was not only glad to see them but also welcomed a break from Arun's moods. He drove us to the neighboring cities of Nice and Monte Carlo, places Mom remembered from summer holidays when she was married to Dad.

She must have noticed the smell of marijuana in the house because on her last day, she expressed concern. She had read that sustained use was linked to paranoia, and while the four of us sat at the dining table, she held up her hand and asked him to promise her to quit. He held her delicate fingers and looked into her eyes. "I promise."

I could tell he had no intention of honoring his promise, and when I questioned him later, he said, "She should have never asked me that."

He had already told me his hierarchy of loves: first Baba, then me, then marijuana. I had scraped above his love of weed. Mom might think she could reason with him, but Arun didn't listen to anyone—other than the elders, and of course, Baba.

For me, his smoking was a relief: without it, he had too many jagged edges.

To pass the time on the weekends, we went to flea markets, and Arun invariably returned with antiques he deemed valuable: marble-topped bedside tables, silver cutlery, a brass angel-shaped lamp. I trusted his instincts and didn't want to halt the only activity he enjoyed. But despite my salary increase, we struggled to make ends meet.

I felt like I had lost my simple mountain man, but then he looked at me with a warm expression and said, "Being with me hasn't changed you, Jo. You're still the innocent girl you were when I met you."

His words validated my efforts. For a moment I was his student again, rising to the challenges of the material world, working to sustain our life together. My morning meditation was my true calling, the place I had discovered thanks to him; it kept me whole. Why would being with him change me?

Three months after our move to Valbonne, Arun announced we needed to leave: there was no future for us there; I should ask Richard to relocate us to the UK. I didn't see how I could make this request so soon after our arrival, so he wrote an email to Richard himself. It was unconventional for a spouse to contact an employee's boss, but Richard read his message, and when I explained that we were unable to settle in the South of France, he agreed to sponsor our move to the UK.

16

ON A KNIFE EDGE

Just before Christmas of 1999, four months after our move to Valbonne, the last of our boxes were delivered into a narrow house in Maidenhead, a town thirty miles west of London. We had exchanged an open-plan house for a small end-of-terrace house with derelict rooms at a higher rent. Cold and wind replaced the mild Mediterranean winter. As Arun ran out to the moving truck—shirtless despite my warning of impending illness—a feeling of hopelessness overtook me, and I heard the words in my mind: *The UK will not be your final destination.*

We spent the holidays alone, sitting on the new navy-blue leather couch Arun had chosen. He had a heavy cold and blew his nose repeatedly. We watched a Bee Gees concert in which Celine Dion joined the band to sing "Immortality." The description of a love beyond the reach of time spoke to me directly.

In contrast to our home, my campus office was bright, my colleagues eager and welcoming. My work had progressed well after the initial headaches, and in January I had to travel to the company headquarters in California where an inside team was developing a new sales commission system. The order of the business hotel, the perfectly made-up bed with crisp white sheets, the breakfast buffet, the walk to work in the sunshine, and the chats with my American colleagues lifted me from the pressures of my home life. And I stepped into Arun's charmed existence in California before his exile to India.

By my second trip in March, Arun put me in contact with a young man he had befriended in prison. He had met Ron in the weightlifting yard and encouraged him to take up Aikido when he got out. Ron not only followed his advice but became a master. I couldn't wait to meet someone from Arun's past who would share firsthand knowledge of his life before Rishikesh. All I knew was what he had told me himself; Ron would flesh out the story.

We made plans to have dinner at a restaurant near my hotel, and he arrived with an older mentor. The two men sat across from me, and we fell into easy conversation. Ron's eyes lit up when he spoke about Arun and how his life had changed since they met. His gratitude and appreciation were palpable, and as we neared the end of the meal, he told me he had been so fascinated by his experience with Arun that he questioned people who had known him in LA.

"Some people thought he was a god. Others said he was a devil."

I wasn't surprised. Arun was charismatic, but not everyone saw beyond his brash persona to the good of his spiritual work. Not even the man responsible for introducing him to his future clients.

Arun met Bikram Choudhury in LA in the late seventies, long before he became famous and copyrighted his hot yoga sequence as Bikram Yoga. Back then, he let Arun sit in a corner of his modest yoga hall and attend classes for free. From his place of observation, Arun came across the elite who would become some of his earliest massage clients and building blocks of his business. Arun described Bikram as a man with a huge ego.

"When I told him he was going too far, he didn't like it. Power went to his head." Distinguishing his own style of influence, he said, "I am a king-maker, not a king."

After some time, the two didn't see eye to eye and parted ways.

While I had been in California, Arun had gone to India and returned with a deal. His son-in-law—the same one we visited with his daughter in Delhi—offered to make him a partner in an attractive agricultural project. He needed twenty-thousand pounds urgently to secure his investment. I was surprised that he had committed the money without consulting with me and without checking that we could obtain a loan, but the prospect of developing an income in India was appealing. Perhaps this was how we would leave our dead-end life in Europe.

Our current bank refused the loan, and Arun was distraught. If we didn't come up with the money in the next few days, the opportunity would be lost. I found another bank more amenable to foreign clients and secured a short-term loan in exchange for our custom. I didn't like seeing him so upset, but equally, he had brought the pressure on himself, then made it my problem.

My trips to California had reminded me of the quality of life in the US, and I longed to move back. I had been away three years and missed my culture and the proximity to Mom and Saby. My vision of Arun with a successful massage business didn't match with how he behaved in the UK, whiling away the afternoons sitting in front of the television, drinking a few bottles of Hobgoblin ale. I knew better than to show concern, but his mood was spiraling down further than in Valbonne. Something had to change.

I hired an American lawyer I had found online. He specialized in complicated immigration cases and would review Arun's case for a reasonable fee, then present his findings over a thirty-minute consultation. On the evening of the meeting, Arun and I huddled over the phone, listening intently to his advice. He spoke gently but firmly and reiterated what we had previously been told: Arun had no chance of returning to the US with his criminal record. "If I were you, I would build your life in Europe."

My belly hollowed at the news; my mind sank into the emptiness of our life. Arun made no comment: there was nothing to say.

THAT SPRING, Mom asked if I could help her find new tenants for her apartment in Paris, a spacious two-bedroom on the eighth floor of a modern building. A balcony ran along the large open-space living room and overlooked the green expanse of the Bois de Boulogne and the cluster of towers at La Défense. The property was in my name, but she had managed it since her divorce, and I never considered it mine

Shortly after we'd been to Paris to show the place to real estate agents, Arun traveled to India again, and when he returned, he had a new ask: one hundred and fifty thousand euros to pay the balance of his agricultural investment. I froze at the sum. He insisted that the deal was good and he didn't want to give up his deposit, but my former enthusiasm about his drive and plans in India turned to anguish. Why did he have to be so rash? And how on earth would I come up with that kind of money?

He mentioned the apartment in Paris, but I didn't understand the connection.

"It's yours."

I corrected him: Mom had raised Saby and me on her own; whatever she earned from the apartment belonged to her.

He dropped the topic but brought up the money he owed

every day. His persistence and anxiety over losing the deal filled our space. I couldn't think of anything else. I understood the requirement to pay for the land but couldn't fathom how he had made a commitment before securing the funds. Living with him felt like a ticking time bomb.

I also knew what he wanted me to do and came up with an idea. Saby had turned eighteen and just graduated from high school. The apartment was currently empty. What if instead of finding a new tenant, we sold it and split the profit between Mom, Saby, and me? Mom, who had benefitted from it until now, would receive an inflow of cash and be free of the hassle of managing a property abroad and finding new tenants.

I called her and shared my thoughts, and to my surprise, she agreed. We met in Paris later that summer, and she selected the pieces of antique furniture she wanted to ship back to New York. They had been in her family or Dad's since they lived in Egypt. I could sell or keep whatever was left. I breathed easier, knowing I had found a solution that worked for everyone.

Back in Maidenhead, we moved out of the dark terraced house to a spacious standalone home close to the town center. The rent would claim close to half my salary, but something had to change: the lack of light and gloomy decor was affecting our mental health.

Tao made an appearance in our new home on a Saturday. He opened a bottle of Hobgoblin and took a sip as diagonal sunrays pierced through the living room windows. His gaze settled on me, and he asked how I was doing. I told him about Arun's investment in India, my hope for a future there, and our plan to sell the apartment.

He set the ale on the coffee table. "Why are you selling it?"

"We need the money."

"Why don't you borrow it?"

I explained my duty to Mom and her need for the money.

"She doesn't need it."

"She's been using it to support us for years."

"She spends like there's no tomorrow. She'll never have enough."

I took a breath, observed the contours of the low inbuilt rock shelf on the opposite wall.

Tao continued. "Did you ever wonder how the apartment came into your hands now?" He paused, light flickering in his eyes. "I've been working hard on the other side. I shouldn't do it, but I care about you."

Was that why he hadn't visited for a while?

"She should have given it to you when you turned eighteen. I corrected the situation."

Tao's caring paternal tone eased the tension I had been feeling, but when he left, I was torn by his suggestion and consulted with Arun. He agreed it was better to keep the apartment and borrow against it.

I wasn't so sure.

Arun kept up the pressure about sending money to India, but I still couldn't bring myself to contact my bank in France and ask for such a large loan. He didn't give up, and finally I spoke with my advisor about it. She had no authority to decide on loans of that amount and scheduled a meeting with the branch director in person.

We made the trip to Fontainebleau and sat in her box office, while a mustachioed man in a dark suit squeezed in beside her. I explained that we wanted the money to build a retirement home in Rishikesh. The agricultural deal had fallen apart, but Arun had reinvested his deposit into a plot of land where we would build our home.

The director listened intently, then said, "I don't like this project of yours. If I were you, I wouldn't do it." He paused and stared into my eyes. "But if you're set on it, I'll approve it. On one condition: you never come back here asking for another loan to invest in India again."

I absorbed his stern warning in silence, not quite believing he had agreed to my request, not wanting to say anything that might change his mind.

A week later, the paperwork to mortgage my apartment was done, and I had the money in my account. With Arun's encouragement and support, I had managed to secure unimaginable funds—just in time to transfer them to India. But I had no idea how I would explain my actions to Mom. Despite Tao's assertions that he had intervened on my behalf, I had betrayed her trust. There was no way to change that fact.

I didn't bring up the topic of the apartment sale until she asked casually how things were going.

I had to come clean. "I decided not to sell it."

"Should I rent it again?"

"I—I'm going to keep it."

"What do you mean, keep it?"

"It's in my name."

"Yes, someday it will be yours."

I murmured, "You should have given it to me when I turned eighteen."

"If you hadn't suggested selling it, I wouldn't have stopped renting it."

I felt selfish, but this was my opportunity to build a life in India. Tao was right: Mom wanted for nothing. She had a luxurious lifestyle on Fifth Avenue and spent without counting. Our conversation ended at an impasse, and I didn't hear from her again for a few days.

Then on Sunday, Dad phoned and spoke to me with strained concern. "Your mother is worried about you."

"Oh yeah?"

"She told me you took the apartment from her."

"It's in my name. I'm twenty-seven now. She should have given it to me when I turned eighteen."

"But it's not yours to take. I bought that apartment."

"Mom's Dad bought it."

"He only paid the deposit. Who do you think paid for the rest? It belongs to me."

"Then why did you entrust it to me?"

"So you could have it someday, but not now."

Dad didn't hold any property in his name. If he had chosen me, it wasn't from care but opportunism.

"You used me, Dad. Then and always."

His tone sharpened. "You're stealing it, Jo. That's all."

My hands trembled on the receiver. "I don't think we have anything more to say to each other."

His voice sent a shiver down my spine. He had sounded confident. Mom hadn't been in touch for a while. What was going on between them?

I had the passwords to their emails and decided to check their accounts. I went upstairs to the computer and started with hers. She still had the same password, and after scrolling through a long list of unread marketing emails, I came to a message from Dad. The subject line was "Intervention." The air hitched in my throat as I read the content. He was telling her about a cult specialist that his business associate, the same woman who had read Arun's case files, had found. They would have a family meeting with him, then decide on their next move. I was also able to access Dad's account and found more personal correspondence with the same woman.

I ran downstairs, where Arun was watching television, and stood next to him. Barely catching a breath, I said, "I can't believe it. How could they?"

He muted the sound and looked up. "What happened?'

"Dad contacted a cult specialist. They're making plans to ambush me. I can't believe them. I hate them both." Warm tears filled my eyes. They had stood by my relationship with Arun when it suited them, but now that I was asserting my legal right, they wanted to prove I was in cult. They were willing to hurt me and ruin my life for money.

I dialed Dad's number. "I never thought you would stoop so low."

"What is it, Jo?"

"I found your e-mails. I know what you're doing."

Through a veneer of calm, tension laced his voice. "You pushed things too far."

"Just because you're not getting your way, you think I'm in a cult?"

"You're not the person we knew, Jo. That's not how we raised you."

I forced myself to slow my speech. "You used me when it suited you. I am not going to let you use me anymore. This ends our relationship right now."

I hung up in sobs.

Arun opened his arms. "Come sit here."

I huddled into his warm body.

"They're upset, that's all. They don't like you standing up for yourself."

My voice quivered. "They have no right."

"Money corrupts people."

I struggled to take full breaths. "They're shallow and materialistic."

He rubbed my back. "You're the only one I care about."

"I won't let them win." I wiped my eyes. "Tomorrow I'll call a lawyer."

17

I'LL DIE HERE

I phoned Marc, the only French lawyer I knew, the following morning. Although he was Dad's lawyer, Dad owed him a large unpaid bill, and I trusted Marc's advice. He sounded unconcerned by my revelation and responded in a measured calm tone. "I wouldn't worry about it. They'll struggle to prove you're not in your right mind."

I didn't worry about my parents' plans again.

Over the Christmas holiday, Arun and I went to Rishikesh and stayed at an ashram in front of the Ganges, close to the plot of land he had bought. It had been over three years since I'd been back, and I relished the return to the peaceful environment we both loved, where I could indulge in my spiritual practice. I noted my meditation experiences in my journal—seeing the elders as black shadows or light tremors from holding my breath and the locks—and shared them all with Arun. He listened with interest and offered new instructions or advice. Here—on the banks of the Ganges, in the shelter of the hills— he was free of the demons that pursued him in Europe.

When he took me to see the plot, an open corner with an open view over the river, I pointed out a small Hindu temple.

"I wanted this for you," he said.

We would have our own place of worship. How did he know me so well? I was overjoyed.

On our return to Delhi, we had dinner at a restaurant with his son-in-law. He knew about the loan against my apartment in Paris, and I told him I was thinking about selling it, repaying the mortgage, and bringing the rest of the money to India.

His face opened into a wide smile, and his eyes bulged with characteristic brightness. "I don't think it's a good idea. Don't sell that place and move the money to India."

He sounded sincere, like he had my best interests in mind despite the benefit to Arun's family if I brought additional funds to India. I weighed my dislike of debt with his conviction and decided to heed his advice. It was an inspired call.

Back in the UK, Arun was as despondent as ever. The developments in India hadn't altered the monotony of his existence; the daily afternoon drinking and naps that transported him to the other side continued as if nothing had changed. We didn't have a car and spent the weekends walking the Maidenhead High Street where he stopped at charity shops, sifted through bric-a-brac and brought home the objects of his fancy. We attended an auction in a neighboring town, and spent significantly more on what he deemed to be valuable antiques. Caught up in his enthusiasm, I joined him in bidding, and we ended up paying for all of it by credit card. When I realized my mistake, I reentered all the lots at the next auction and made up for some of the loss.

I suggested to Arun that we move to India—there was nothing for us in the UK—but he questioned my logic. "What will you do there?"

"I don't know. Teach, I guess."

"What will you teach?"

"Excel?"

He wasn't convinced, but I was at a loss.

I took comfort in his continued focus on yoga. He spoke often about the true practice that led to a clear mind and a better life. He also wrote his thoughts. "All problems in life are our own creations. We create them because of greed, selfishness, by lying or various disturbing thoughts." His words and teaching inspired me to keep striving for the golden state of enlightenment.

But in everyday life his only diversion seemed to be buying objects. When he discovered a jeweler in the neighboring town of Windsor, he was excited to take me there and show me a unique woman's antique watch. It was dainty and impractical: a diamond-studded dial with daisies inlaid with precious stones on either end and gold-corded straps. But once again, I couldn't resist the pull of his enthusiasm; when he asked if I wanted it, I took out my credit card.

He decided he wanted a solid platinum chain for himself, and we returned to the jeweler. The man smiled in surprise at the request. He didn't have such an item but could fashion a bespoke piece if we brought him the metal. Arun agreed. Then the jeweler asked if he realized how heavy the chain would be. Arun didn't mind; he liked the idea that no one would realize it wasn't steel. We bought the raw platinum in London at a monumental cost. By our second summer in the UK, I was promoted to senior manager, but my salary barely kept up with his wants.

I tried to interest him in teaching a local group yoga class, and though we set up a website and rented a community hall, he gave up after the first orientation session: only a handful of people had shown up, and it wasn't worth his time.

I finally suggested that he volunteer at one of the charity shops he enjoyed so much. He agreed, probably to appease me, and returned from his first day with a down duvet that couldn't be sold. By his second day, he quit—or was let go. He said the elderly white women who worked there didn't like him and had reprimanded him for stuffing his pockets with donations. I was so despondent at the quick end of his voluntary work that I didn't even pause to think about what he had done, how he had brought it upon himself.

On 9/11, he was sitting at home watching television when the Twin Towers were blown up. He greeted me with the shocking news on my return from work, and along with the rest of the world, I reeled at the loss of life and massive destruction in my city. Helpless and far from home, I felt a surge of desire to return and be with my family.

Shortly after, on a weekend afternoon, while we were sitting on the navy leather couch, Arun said, "I'll die if I stay here. I want to go back to Paris as soon as possible."

Though I lived with him and knew how restless and desperate he was, he had never used such strong language. But we had tried Paris already: would he really be happy there?

He was sure of it, and recalled how when he was deported from the US, the elders had told him he would someday live in Paris. He hadn't believed them then, but now realized they were right.

I brought up the subject of relocation with my North American manager, citing personal reasons this time, as it didn't make sense from the business point of view for me to move back to France. I said I would pay for my own move but would need the company to offer me a French contract and sponsor my work visa.

She heard me out and agreed, but retracted her offer after I questioned my salary conversion. I couldn't believe my stroke of bad luck, and Arun wasn't understanding about the setback. He reiterated his hopelessness about life and pushed me to make alternative immigration plans with Marc, the French lawyer. I felt Arun's sense of urgency, but even if Mark helped us get back into the country, we weren't going anywhere without my job.

When it seemed like the original deal couldn't be salvaged,

I called on a senior HR colleague who had also become a friend. I explained what had happened with my boss, shared Arun's state of despair, and confided in her something I hadn't even admitted to myself. "I think he might ask for a divorce if we don't move as planned."

She listened without speaking, then said, "Leave it with me."

Three months later, we were back in Dad's studio.

WE HIRED a contractor to give Dad's place a makeover: replace the withered carpet with laminate flooring; remove the tired wallpapers; and paint the walls the apricot swami color. Our belongings filled the space: clothing on an open double-tiered rack, books behind the crystal doors of a bureau bookcase. On the floor: a low square Japanese tea table, and handwoven wool Tibetan carpets Arun had brought from India—his navy blue, mine tomato red—that had traveled with us everywhere. I sat on the blue one and read by the window.

It took me a few days to stop hearing the street noise outside Dad's studio as I fell asleep, but within a week it felt like we had never left, and I put our dim days in the UK behind me. I had my job, and Arun was communicating with Surat on the construction of our house in Rishikesh. Dad and I had reached a truce. After our confrontation over his planned cult intervention, he had backed down, and though he didn't initiate phone conversations, he answered my calls and agreed to let us stay in his studio for a while. As Paris glowed in spring light, and sunshine poured in from the south-facing door window, I felt at peace; buoyed by our return, confident that the worst was behind us.

PART III

THE YOGA SCHOOL

18

OUR PLACE

I first met Gabriel in my apartment just before we rented it out to cover the mortgage. He was a young man who taught yoga in the city and had been introduced to Arun by the drug dealer. Marveling at her ability to connect people, Arun had told me, "She doesn't do anything herself, but she's a magnet who brings people together."

Gabriel's eyes shone with kindness, and he greeted me with a beatific smile. Dark wavy hair softened the angles of his face. He stood up and proffered a hand adorned with silver rings, wrists wrapped in leather bracelets. Pendants hung from his neck. I shook his hand, noticed his skull ring, and took an immediate liking to him.

Arun sat on the opposite end of the L-shaped couch and looked at him with pride. "Gabriel teaches yoga every Saturday. His class is always full."

The young protégé listened with quiet luminosity.

He soon made regular visits to our studio when Arun invited him for lunch on Saturdays. The three of us sat on the floor at the Japanese table and ate the spicy dahl and rice Arun had prepared in the closet kitchen. When we were done,

Gabriel rose without a word, gathered the empty dishes, and washed them under a trickle of water. He was twenty-five and moved with unencumbered grace. I had turned twenty-nine but felt much older.

Arun took him under his wing and initiated him into the practice Agni Yoga, how to cultivate the body's inner heat for health and longevity. Gabriel, in turn, invited him to teach his bohemian friends at a loft where they met on the other side of the city. Arun brought bamboo poles from home and led them into the spine stretches, forward-bends, squats, and lunges. The practice appealed to them, and for the first time since he had left India five years earlier, he had a following. The drug dealer had made a fortuitous connection, indeed.

As THE MONTHS WENT BY, Arun spoke with Surat in increasingly vociferous tones. I gathered from the Hindi I had picked up over the years that there were issues with the build. After one of these heated conversations, Arun said we'd need another fifty thousand euros. My chest tightened. How could we be in the same predicament again so soon? He spoke about material cost overruns, but I had only one question. "Are you sure that's all we need?"

He held up his hands, palms facing me, and shook his head. "This is it. The foundations and walls are there. All we need now is paint and tiles."

I ignored my bank director's earlier warning and started with him. He hadn't changed his mind: "I already told you not to come back asking for more money to invest in India. I will not do it."

Undeterred, I found another bank in our neighborhood and met an advisor there. After reviewing my salary slips and property documents in his glass cubicle, the young associate approved the mortgage on the spot. I was making a very good living by French standards. He didn't ask about other liabilities on the apartment, and I didn't offer the information.

Around the same time, Arun saw a listing in the paper for a small studio apartment for sale in the area and suggested we buy it as an investment. The price was attractive, and his plan made sense. The same bank offered us a full loan with no deposit. All these investments meant that I had very little to spend on myself, but I was securing my future. I was also lucky that Mom generously bought me clothes whenever I returned to New York. The fact that I had taken possession of the apartment still loomed between us, but after an initial discussion, she had dropped the subject. Even Saby had commented, "I can see it both ways."

Arun traveled to Rishikesh ahead of me that summer. It was the first time in four years that we'd spend a couple of months apart, and though I missed him, I relished the uninterrupted hours reading by the window. I still sought knowledge from books, and with time to concentrate, I made my way through *Vasistha's Yoga*, a seven-hundred-page philosophical text.

When I joined him in August, I finally discovered the place he had been building for over a year: a large L-shaped single-story brick house in an otherwise modest neighborhood. The master bedroom was huge—twice the size of our studio apartment in Paris, a king-sized mahogany bed was framed in a cement alcove on the far wall. He had bought a thick hotel-quality spring mattress: the best he could find. Beyond the adjoining dressing room was a bathroom large enough to fit a round spa bath and a wide glass sink with crystal fittings. Despite rooftop solar panels, when I tried to fill the bath, only lukewarm water flowed. On the other side of the L, were the kitchen, smaller living room, and second bedroom.

He had spared no expense: shiny floor tiles in the master bedroom suite; marble flooring through the rest of the house; modern kitchen furnishings and granite countertops.

"It's not what I wanted," Arun commented on the dispro-portionate layout, "but Surat didn't understand me."

"It's really nice," I said.

From the roof I contemplated the curve of the majestic river against the backdrop of the Himalayan foothills, an awe-inspiring panoramic view that alone justified our significant investment.

Now that our house was built, I could see that the temple I had noticed on my last visit was outside our boundary wall. Had I misunderstood Arun when he said it was ours? I wanted to ask him about it, but he had done so much with the house I let it go.

One afternoon, close to the end of my visit, he sat cross-legged on the bed with his back straight. I was by his side, and he brought up the widow who had been our former neighbor at the mountain house. "She asked me when I would marry her." His eyes searched mine.

My jaw dropped. "Where did she get that?"

He shrugged. "I don't know."

"Doesn't she know you're married to me?"

The widow's question was too preposterous to consider. How could she possibly interpret Arun's kindness as romantic interest, let alone a marriage offer? She was only a poor, attrac-tive woman on whom he had taken pity.

The sweltering humidity of the monsoon weighed the daylight hours, but by evening a breeze rose from the river and night-blooming jasmine infused the air. Sitting on the veranda, Arun and I might exchange a word or two, but it wasn't neces-sary to speak then; it was enough to listen to the trill of the crickets and take in the night. Someday I would retire from corporate work, and we would come home to this unparalleled natural beauty. We would live simply in Europe to have luxury in India. We had found each other again, and our shared mission had been restored: everything would be better from now on.

During his time in Rishikesh, Arun had invented a new set of exercises, inspired by an electrical board cover left lying on the patio. He stood on the low wooden structure, bent from the waist, and grabbed hold of its front edge. As he pulled himself down, his spine lengthened. That first move spawned a series of assisted standing and seated forward bends. He called it simply "board exercises," and on our return to Paris, we practiced together in the small space of our studio.

As he had instructed, I sat behind the board, propped one heel on top of it, and stretched forward so my hands reached the edge. My spine curved like a bow over my leg, and he commented, "Not very flexible for the wife of a yoga teacher."

Embarrassed by his assessment, I tugged harder to reduce the gap between my torso and my legs. I thought of myself as his top student, worthy of being his mate, and didn't want to be seen wanting in any way.

IN THE MONTHS since we met, Gabriel became interwoven into our lives. He ate lunch with us every Saturday and felt like Arun's adopted son, our chosen family. Our conversation invariably turned to our yoga ambitions, and their connection seemed destined for more.

"Why don't you start a yoga school together?" I asked Arun one afternoon after Gabriel had left.

His answer was quick. "The elders won't let me teach in public."

I was aware that the secret practice could only be handed down from teacher to student, as it had over the centuries, but what about the physical exercises? Surely he could teach those more broadly?

By September, Gabriel had found a slot at a martial arts studio for Arun to teach his exercises in the early morning. It was his preferred time of day to practice and seemed like an ideal opportunity. I designed a flyer to advertise the classes, including Gabriel's drawing of a lotus-sitting figure reminiscent of the youthful Babaji. Perhaps this was how we would introduce Agni Yoga to the world. We named our new venture City Yoga.

After a few weeks, Arun only had a few students, and he asked the owner for another slot later in the day. None was available, so he decided to quit; he didn't want to work only to cover the cost of the hall. I had been attending his classes on the days I worked from home, and though I understood his reasoning, I was disappointed by how quickly he gave up. Building a student base would take time.

I returned to my earlier vision—a center dedicated to Agni Yoga—and renewed my ask: "Can we open our own school?"

His answer was the same: the elders hadn't approved.

Somehow I didn't lose hope and felt sure it was only a matter of time for the elders to review their decision. Someday Arun would be guiding students into a deep practice; Gabriel at his side, teaching his own classes; clients filling our hall. The future was ours to create.

The next time I asked, Arun confirmed that the elders had relented and finally given us their blessing. I wasn't surprised: I was elated. The idea of opening our own school was the crowning moment of my seven years with Arun; a return to the bliss of our early relationship in Rishikesh; the end of our trials in Europe. Not only would the school give him a sense of personal purpose, but we would also contribute to improving the world. We couldn't keep the mental and physical benefits for ourselves; we would share his unique teaching. Not its details, but its peace.

· · ·

ARUN WANTED a space in the commercial district around the Champs Élysées, where rents were exorbitant. After viewing an office for six-thousand euros a month, I found an internet listing for a ground-floor unit close by. The cobbled floor would need to be cemented, but the place already had two washrooms and a small room behind them which we could use for massage. It had wide-open areas and a high glass ceiling at the back. The rent of forty-eight hundred euros seemed more reasonable, and based on my business plan, we would need an average of seven students per class to cover our expenses: well within our growth projections. We made our decision on the spot.

The property agent offered us a rent-free period of six months in exchange for completing the renovations, including building two changing rooms with showers. His only additional requirement was a personal guarantee since we had no prior business record. It was risky to tie my personal assets to the business, but I had to cross this hurdle to bring our dream to life.

We signed the lease at his office, and after he congratulated us with a grin on his face, he offered to open a bottle of champagne. We thanked him and declined, then stepped out into a cold December afternoon.

I wanted to give Gabriel the news right away and asked Arun to phone him then and there. They exchanged a few words, then their conversation came to a quick end.

"What happened?" I asked.

"He sounded groggy. I think I woke him up."

I looked at my watch: it was past noon. "Didn't he know we were signing today?" I had imagined him waiting for our call, anxious for the news, ready to meet us at the new place.

Arun shrugged. "Must have had a late night."

Gabriel's reaction didn't stack. We held the keys to a significant new business where we would soon start major renovations, yet our partner seemed uninterested in joining our celebration and making plans. A sense of foreboding flashed through my mind—had we misread him? Did he not care that much about our shared venture? But I couldn't linger in those thoughts. I had bet my personal assets on City Yoga's success and needed to focus on the work ahead. Gabriel was probably laid-back, that was all. Once he saw the place, it would spark his dormant enthusiasm.

Arun found a Pakistani builder in the local French-English magazine and hired him, happy to speak with him in their common language. Within two weeks, the cement floor was laid, and the changing rooms with showers had been built. Then when it was time to move on to the internal work—laying floor tiles and painting the walls—the builder and his team were nowhere to be found. Arun spent hours shouting over the phone about the problems he was causing.

I had poured all of my savings—fifty-thousand euros—into the renovations, but we still ran out of funds, and I applied for a short-term bank loan to complete the work. When I spoke with Dad about our plans and the loan I had secured for an additional twenty-five thousand euros, he said, "I can lend you the money. Don't borrow it."

His thoughtfulness and unexpected offer stunned me. After all we had been through around Arun and our recent fight over the apartment, I never expected him to take an interest in my project. "Thank you, Dad. I'll pay you back as soon as possible."

We finally opened the doors to City Yoga, which we called the school, on the last Monday in January, a little over a year after moving from the UK.

Gabriel taught the maiden class. He was wearing a ribbed undershirt and loose cotton trousers. All in white, his wiry arms bare, he led a small group of students, including me. The floor of the hall was covered in teal judo mats, which Arun had insisted on as the signature feature of our method, a nod to his martial arts past. Light poured in from the steepled glass ceiling as Gabriel started with a few elements of Agni Yoga, then moved on to the set Ashtanga sequence he had first learned.

At the end, we all sat on the floor in front of him, and he gathered his hands in prayer, casting his beatific smile upon us. A light breeze filtered through gaps in the ceiling windows. Pigeons pecked the glass, and a chorus of children sounded from a nearby school. As my breath moved in and out of my body, my mind dwelled in the peace of the moment. We did it. We had actually opened our own school.

From that day on, Arun and I went to City Yoga every morning by seven, opened the carriage doors, and burned a stick of Indian incense. The sweet penetrating scent permeated the air and bridged the inner space of the school with the outside world. He had chosen orange-yellow floor tiles and apricot paint for the reception area. We had a desk and bookshelf by the back wall, and an Indonesian-style teak bench in the center of the reception area. The place conveyed the cheerfulness of an elementary school paired with a touch of eastern artistry.

When we had been open a week, as we stood by the main entrance looking onto the street, I asked him, "How long do you think we'll be here?"

Hands in his jeans pockets, he gazed in the clear daylight. "Nine years. Eighteen, twenty-seven. As long as this building stands, City Yoga will be here."

19

THE WOMAN IN BLACK

On a Sunday afternoon in February, I sat at the desk waiting for students to arrive for the introductory class which we offered once a week to attract new clients. Gabriel, the usual instructor, was warming up in the hall. With thirty minutes to go, there wasn't much to do, and I arranged the registration forms in a neat pile. The reception area was quiet, the smell of incense in the air. It was that moment of anticipation before new faces came in, new clients to welcome and sign up. Then the glass door opened, and I looked up. A woman dressed completely in black crossed the threshold. Her skin was pale, and a few wispy strands of hair, neither brown nor blond, escaped from her tight bun. She directed her gaze beyond me, as if expecting someone else to emerge, then seeing no one, she took a few furtive steps toward the desk. She paused, still searching, then turned to me. "I'm Angela. I'm a friend of Gabriel." Her eyes looked like the ocean before a storm.

I put on an open smile. "He's preparing at the back."

Her lips parted, and a look of concern crossed her face. "He told me to meet him here."

I pointed to the hall behind me to reassure her. "You can go ahead."

She clutched her bulging tote bag and walked away, but I couldn't let go of her so soon. Her attire was striking—a black skirt falling in folds below the knee and a tight black jacket—but that wasn't it. It was her energy: fearful, palpable and cloying.

I left the desk to see if she needed anything and found her standing by the open door of the hall. Gabriel smiled when he saw me, but when she sensed my presence, she shrank back.

"Is everything okay?" I asked.

She nodded.

I showed her the door to the women's changing room, and she scurried toward it, as if following an instruction I hadn't meant to give.

New students arrived, and I focused on checking them in, but once the class started and I was sitting alone, I thought about this woman's seeming reluctance to engage with me. What did she fear?

In the middle of class, I went to peek into the hall from the open door. The class was at capacity, with a student on every mat. Gabriel called out instructions from the front while everyone looked at him and followed. Over twenty people were seated on the floor, one heel up on the board, the other leg bent toward the raised knee. Arms extended toward the board and spines pulled forward, heads dropping to the knees. Some could hold the board, while others placed their hands on the floor. I quickly spotted Angela at the back. Her fingers held the edge, her elbows bent comfortably to the floor. Her torso folded over her legs with the grace of a swan. She easily stood out from the rest of the crowd.

After class when everyone was gone and only Gabriel, Arun, and I remained, Arun asked him, "Who was that woman at the back?"

"You mean Angela? She's the one I told you about."

"The one who does massage?"

"Yeah, she's looking for work. I told her to come today."

"Send her to my morning class."

When we walked home that evening, I said to Arun, "That woman was strange."

"Why do you say that?"

I frowned in the darkness. "I don't know. She was dressed all in black, and she didn't smile. Not even once."

ANGELA RETURNED a couple of days later to take Arun's early morning class. There was only one other woman there, a regular from the martial arts studio who had followed us to our new location. While we were in the one-legged downward dog split, I glanced in their direction. Angela had her palms and one foot pressed into the floor, and her other leg pointed directly to the ceiling. Her back sloped like a hammock. The other woman was performing the position correctly, her back and leg in a diagonal line, but with visible effort. She was assiduous and wanted to develop into a yoga instructor, but she was no match for Angela's precision and seemingly effortless movement.

The four of us gathered in the reception area after class, and Arun commented on Angela's physical skill. The other woman looked on, hoping for an opening to speak with him, but he hardly acknowledged her presence. Angela smiled with genuine warmth and told us about moving to Paris from her native Portugal a couple of years earlier. She lamented the recent loss of her massage job, and Arun didn't miss a beat. "Why don't you work with us?"

Her eyes opened wide. "You need someone now?"

He nodded. "We'll try you out on Jo. If she likes your work, you're hired."

The other woman, who had been listening from a polite distance, left with a quiet smile. Arun dismissed her with a wave, and though I felt sorry he hadn't given her any attention, he clearly had a plan, and I followed his cues. I don't think the other woman ever returned.

Angela gazed from Arun to me, her eyes lit with hope. "I can't believe I met you. You're both such beautiful people."

She sounded genuine—yet so innocent.

After she left, Arun mimicked her mellifluous tone. "You're both beautiful people."

I smiled. "She's sweet."

She was twenty-six, the same age as Gabriel; to my thirty, they both seemed young.

Soon after, Angela traveled to Portugal to visit her family. She apologized for her timing, but it was understandable that she had made other commitments before meeting us. She returned with local gifts for me, I thanked her for her thoughtfulness, knowing any additional expense would be a strain for her.

"You're the one who has been kind," she said.

Her initial reticence had given way to Mediterranean warmth. Whatever snaking fear had enveloped her on her first visit was gone.

Arun took a paternal interest in her personal improvement and suggested lighter-colored work clothes. When he noticed mascara clumped on her lashes, he gave her twenty euros to buy a better one. He always seemed to know what women needed in a way that wouldn't have occurred to me.

And he set the rules: Angela would only massage women; he would handle the men. He added that I wasn't allowed to massage at all, though I wasn't sure why he bothered to say it, since I wasn't trained in massage and showed no inclination for it. Coming from him, these conditions were sacred laws, not practical statements.

Angela transformed the back room into a massage haven. She made her own oils with the sharp scents of rosemary and geranium. I tried out her technique and was sure she would find a loyal clientele. Once she started working with us, it felt like she had been sent to us and was meant to be there to complete our team.

Arun encouraged both Gabriel and her to attend his early morning class, but only Angela did so. She delighted in being able to exercise at her place of work and develop her knowledge of Agni Yoga. She stayed on for her massage appointments, and with her welcoming presence and her knowledge of French, she soon contributed to the reception work. Gabriel taught in the evenings and was rarely awake early enough to attend Arun's morning class, but his absence wasn't just down to his schedule. He respected Arun as a yoga guru, but continued to teach the Ashtanga Yoga in which he had been trained. Arun didn't seem to mind, other than forbidding the practice of the headstand, which he deemed too risky for the neck. Gabriel was unconvinced, but Arun wouldn't bend on that point.

After Arun's morning class, a coterie of women flocked around his desk to ask a question or find a reason to speak with him. On the days I was there, I looked on from a distance, proud that my husband still commanded so much attention at the age of sixty-three.

I spent all my free time working at City Yoga. In the evenings after work and on the weekends, I sat at reception, updating the website I had created, designing ads, printing flyers, keeping up with bookkeeping. The school was my vocation, and every hour I spent there would bring me closer to leaving corporate life.

Gabriel and Angela lived far from the school, and once we settled into a regular work rhythm, Arun suggested that Gabriel move closer. I couldn't imagine him leaving his bohemian neighborhood for a studio on a sleepy residential street, but to my surprise, he agreed. He would cover the rent, and I gave my personal guarantee to secure the lease.

Then Arun turned his attention to Angela and asked me if I wanted her to live with us.

We were still living at Dad's studio and needed to save money while building the business. "Where?"

"We could move somewhere."

I shook my head. She might have filled a gap, both in the business and in our lives, but I didn't want to live with her.

"I thought you might want to keep her close."

Was he implying we should adopt her? She might be young, eager, and compliant, and I felt protective over her, but she was a grown woman. "I don't want to live with anyone other than my husband." He could be creative in his thinking, and I needed to root out his errant notion.

Then he suggested we let her stay at our investment studio. We had left it empty in case Dad ever needed it for his guests. If Angela moved there, she could live close by, and the apartment would be a way of repaying her for the reception work she had taken on. We didn't formalize the terms of the exchange. She spent so many hours at the school anyway, and already felt more like a family member than a coworker. To fix a number to her devotion felt awkward.

When she saw the place, she could hardly believe her luck. To make it hers, Arun offered to have the walls painted the color of her choice. I found the expense excessive, but once again, he was the more thoughtful one.

One morning, while Angela and I were sitting together at the desk, sipping our coffees after class, she took hold of my left hand in both of hers and said, "Will you marry me?"

Her eyes were lit with exuberance, and though I was sure she was joking, I withdrew my hand. "No, I'm already married."

Her gesture had been playful, an expression of her affection, but she needed to know where my loyalty lay.

Angela replaced Gabriel at our Saturday lunches. He had a rich life of his own with friends and activities, but she entered our space willingly and wholeheartedly as no one had before. Such closeness felt predestined, and I asked Arun a question to which I already sensed the answer. "Did we know each other in a past life?"

He looked at me with a grave expression. "You were very close."

Was he implying we had been lovers? I enjoyed her company but didn't feel any sexual attraction. My closest child-hood friends had struggled to accept my relationship with Arun, and his years of drinking and variable moods had been trying. I missed having a close friendship with a woman, and though Angela felt young and needy, she accepted both Arun and me and seemed to have a calming effect on him.

One Saturday, before she arrived, he asked me whether I wanted to give her a piece of jewelry, as a mark of friendship. I didn't specifically recollect my past with Angela, but his suggestion of generosity made sense. Mom had given me pieces from her own mother over the years, and with Arun's love of gold, I had others from India.

"What should I give her?"

"Whatever you want."

I chose a gold chain with a heart-shaped pendant inlaid with diamonds from Mom, and deep-yellow Indian earrings and bangles.

After lunch, with the three of us sitting on the floor, I gave her the gifts in small boxes. Her grey eyes shone as she opened them. She looked up and said, "You are my real family."

20

KNOT

Soon after Angela joined us, Arun asked me to teach her the secret practice. He felt the details would be better explained by a woman. I understood what he meant. To explain the position of the pelvic lock, he would need to locate the perineum between the vagina and anus and might not want to be that explicit with her. Still, I wasn't keen. Despite my eight years of practice and hours spent on the daily hypnotic ritual of focused breathing, I felt unprepared to transmit what he had taught me. I knew the physical details: keeping my spine straight, extending my neck forward, drawing my chin down, holding my breath for a set number of counts, whether full or empty of air. I had experienced subtle physical flutters and heat from the effort of the locks. I had trained my mind to go blank. But the realm of magic eluded me. I hadn't remembered my past life or left my physical body. I hadn't levitated.

I told Arun I wasn't ready.

He insisted. "You know everything there is to know."

I had followed his changing instructions meticulously over the years but struggled to recall my earliest lessons. Taken by the wonders of learning, I had only jotted down key points later. I made no preparations before my first lesson with Angela and hoped the flow of the moment would guide me.

We met in the yoga hall on a Saturday morning. She was already sitting in the lotus pose in the back corner when I arrived, her feet fixed on opposite thighs, her gaze turned inward. Daylight penetrated through the glass ceiling on the other side of her room, but her corner was dim. There were few external street sounds at this time of the day, and the space resonated with emptiness. I sat diagonally from her, across an invisible barrier.

"Arun asked me to teach you."

Her face lifted, her eyes fixed mine. "I know."

Transfixed by the thrum of silence, I couldn't think how to start and realized too late I needed a lesson plan. Without preamble, I explained about the pelvic lock, but when she said she already knew it I was unnerved. I moved on to the slow controlled breathing through the nose, and though she listened intently, my words sounded lifeless.

I showed her how to sit in *siddhasana* with her pelvic floor pressed into her left heel. She found it uncomfortable, adjusted her position several times, then bent her head, and started the slow breathing. I watched for a few moments, but my presence felt like an intrusion, and I closed my eyes and breathed through my rapid heartbeat. How long should I wait? How had Arun managed to teach with attention for days when I struggled on the first?

I instructed her to continue on her own and left the room, sliding the door shut behind me. A surge of relief washed over me when I joined Arun sitting at the computer in the bright fluorescent lights. He asked me how it went.

"Alright, I guess."

Later when we were at home, I said, "I don't think she wants to learn from me."

"Don't say that."

It was true: my first attempt had felt like a failure.

He urged me to try again, but as soon as we were alone together in the silence of the yoga hall, apprehension gripped me. How had Arun made each element of the practice feel important and sacred? In my voice, the instructions sounded banal.

After a stretch of breathing, I asked her how she felt. As she released her right ankle from her left thigh, her eyes bore into mine. "You don't seem comfortable teaching me."

"It's my first time. I'm not sure where to start."

I felt like I had been tested and found wanting.

I told Arun he had to take over teaching Angela, but he made a different suggestion. "Why don't you stay at her place once a week and practice together in the morning? Sit next to her and hold her right hand in your left one. She'll learn directly from you."

At first, I resisted the idea of leaving my home and husband once a week, but he encouraged me to give it a try, only for some time. "It will be good for both of you."

Angela didn't have many friends in Paris, and she cut off whatever contacts she had when she met us. The school became her new home, Arun and I her chosen family. She did mention one close friend, but the friendship had broken off when this woman made a negative comment about Angela's energy. Although I had picked up something troubling the first day she walked into the school, I understood her reaction. A good friend should try to help, and perhaps this is what Arun expected me to do.

I went to her apartment one evening and sat on the futon folded up into a couch. A breeze filtered between the windows at the opposite ends of the studio, and I picked up a sweet scent I couldn't name. "Orange blossom," she said. Ah yes, the smell was deep in my childhood memories: Mom dabbing her face with orange blossom water in bed at the end of the day. I had found it sharp then, but here it felt comforting and clean.

Angela prepared a tasty meal, and while eating, we chatted a bit about her family. She didn't say much, but I sensed that she was glad to be away from her native country, building her own life in Paris. When it came time to sleep, she opened the couch into a double bed and I lay by her side. It felt like a childhood sleepover, and though I hadn't settled easily in other children's homes I fell asleep quickly.

I woke up feeling refreshed. Arun insisted on holding me, or being held, throughout the night. Under the weight of his arm or leg, I experienced vivid, often draining, dreams. I attributed these nightly visions to spirit travel, but without his hold I felt lighter.

We sat for meditation and held hands as instructed. I inhaled slowly and consciously, paused, then exhaled fully. Aware of my responsibility to her, I entered a state of heightened concentration.

Later, when Arun asked if I had felt anything different practicing with her, I said, "Not really. It's nice to be with someone else, but we're really quite different, you know."

"No one said you have to be the same."

"She seems happy in her own little space."

WHEN ANGELA first moved into the studio, he gave her a two-inch brass statue of his chosen deity, the elephant-headed god, Ganesh. The idol had been a gift to me, but I didn't mind when he passed it on to Angela. He had brought a much larger heavy statue that we placed on the top shelf of the bureau bookcase. Besides, he said he could observe Angela in her studio through the figurine. I didn't stop to ask him how: his intentions and abilities were a mystery.

One Saturday before Angela arrived for lunch, I was

contemplating the books in the bookcase, something I enjoyed doing, when Arun stood by me and said, "You know that story about the scholar who went to find Gourd Immortal?" He paused. "It's about Tao. We were amazed when you showed it to us."

I had been fascinated by the scholar who traveled in the mountains to seek enlightenment, his journey a mirror of my own, but our connection was even deeper. I had recognized him on an unconscious level. Arun's revelation stunned me. But he didn't stop there. His expression turned serious. "The author didn't get the whole story. There's an important part missing. Tao married one of Gourd Immortal's daughters."

I frowned.

Arun looked at me expectantly.

As his words settled in my mind, the realization struck my belly, and I looked into his eyes. "Angela's not ...?"

He nodded.

Angela, drawn to us from the past, had been Tao's wife and my sister-in-law. Tao only appeared through Arun. The implication of what Arun had revealed was damning. Would they seek to be lovers again in this life? In that one revelation, the peaceful waters on which I had been navigating opened into a dark vortex below.

"What are we going to do now?"

"Nothing you don't want to."

When Tao appeared later after Angela had arrived, I observed their behavior. He was cheerful and gentle as always, and she came to his side and looked up at him with fondness. She was respectful and familiar; no hint of apprehension crossed her gaze as she interacted with the spirit who came through my husband's body. Arun must have shared the same news with her, but I had no idea when.

Once our common past, and her former relationship with Tao, was out in the open, Arun shared with us how he had recognized Angela: when he went to touch her hips to correct her position on the first day she came to take the free class, she had taken his hands and placed them on his belly. I was appalled by the intimacy of her gesture, but she had no memory of it. Arun was sure, and I felt trapped.

Tao visited every Saturday with clockwork regularity. Reunited with his lost love, he wanted to see her as much as possible. Each time we visited a different neighborhood; he accompanied us to the Bastille Place or the Luxembourg Gardens with a delight unknown to Arun. He reveled in the late spring sunshine, the light which he said was absent on the other side. His joy was contagious, and I relaxed in his presence, confident that my earlier apprehension had been unfounded. My brother would never hurt me: despite the sacrifice, his relationship would remain platonic.

Then one afternoon, as we were walking back after an outing, we reached the intersection where Angela would turn up the street to her place, and Tao and I would go in the opposite direction. But instead of joining me, he started to walk up the street toward Angela's apartment. As if he'd had an afterthought, he said, "I'm going with her."

Nothing more. His certainty bumped up to my shock so strongly that no words came to me.

Angela, who was walking with him, turned back for a moment and looked at me with a silent stare, an apology for what they were about to do—as if she wished it could have been otherwise. But it only lasted an instant. She hurried her steps until she caught up with him.

He never looked back.

I stood frozen on the pavement and watched them for a few moments until they became distant images. I wished I'd had a line to reel in Tao back to me. I wanted to say: no. You can't do this; I won't allow it. If I could have done anything to stop them,

I would have. But it was too late. Only the shining specks of mica on the pavement met my gaze.

I trudged home through a wall of grief. I threw myself on the bed in the empty studio and succumbed to howls of pain. When I came up for air, the walls closed in on me. I wanted to be anywhere but there. The moment when Tao walked away with Angela played on repeat in my mind. With each vision a fresh lash gripped my throat; the sting of shame and abandonment clung to my skin. I heaved and gulped for air as if life was being sucked out of me. Arun had been taken from me, and I had been left on the side of the road. I lay awake and sank into an abyss with no exit.

At the first grey light of dawn, my mind started to emerge from the depths. By five-thirty I called Angela to ask if Arun had returned. She answered in a whisper, "Not yet. I'll call you as soon as he returns." She sounded caring, and I felt less alone.

When Arun's key turned in the door just after six, I was sitting at the dining table drinking coffee. "Arun, is it you?"

"Yes."

"I've been waiting."

He sat across from me, his large hands pressed into the table, and peered into my face. "Are you all right? Tao was worried."

"It was hard." How could I express the crush of abandonment, the cloying sting of shame? "I'll make more coffee."

I stood at the counter, glad for something to do, and gathered my thoughts. Sunlight filtered into the room. I placed his cup on the table and exhaled through my tight belly.

"What if . . . what if I can't take it?"

He looked at me with concern. "Then I won't let it happen again."

"What about Tao?"

"He'll stop coming."

"He'll never visit?"

"No. It would be too painful for him."

I could put an end to their relationship now, lose my brother and Angela, two people who cared about me, and return to the volatile side of Arun. Or I could accept an impossible situation.

Our crowded space looked identical to the day before, but our lives had changed inexorably. I had believed that Arun and I were linked by an extraordinary love; that despite his drinking and outbursts, he would someday return to me healed. But in the seconds when Tao walked away with Angela, my world collapsed.

When he and I first became lovers, he had likened a close relationship between two people to a smooth thread. Once broken, it can be tied back together, but when you run your fingers over it, you will always feel the knot. That's how I felt now. A knot had formed at the core of my being. I would do my best to ignore it, but I would never stop feeling it. I knew—even if I couldn't admit it consciously—that the breach was too deep.

Sometimes you die but you don't leave.

21

BLOOD IS THICKER THAN WATER

A ngela visited us frequently even when Tao wasn't around. She was close to both Arun and me, and now that she was married to my brother, I felt an added sense of responsibility for her. When Tao visited on Saturdays, we spent the day together, and he left with her in the early evening. I had recovered from the initial shock and devastation, but a surge of anxiety rose when I found myself alone. I tuned into episodes of *Friends* and distracted myself with the characters' humorous exchanges and everyday situations. I escaped my life through a parallel world in New York City.

Sometime after we moved from the UK to Paris, but before we had the school, Arun had spoken to me seriously one day about our relationship. I could tell from his expression that he would say something important. Would he bring up our sexual estrangement again? I still watched myself around him, sensitive to his moods, aware of my own failings.

"Some women need another woman. To help the couple come back together."

I listened to his words. He was implying a lesbian relationship, a female companion for me, and though the years with him had been lonely, distanced from my own friends, I couldn't imagine another woman with us. And what kind of person would willingly enter the sphere of a married couple? What kind of woman would engage in selfless subservience? No, this was not what I wanted. It wasn't what I felt I needed.

Now that Angela was in our life I wondered—though she was Tao's wife, and Tao was distinct from Arun—whether he had been alluding to a convenient merging of these complicated relationships. But whatever he had in mind, I would never accept it. I might make a concession for Tao—for whatever bond held me to him from the past—but I would never share Arun with anyone.

At the school, in our public life, no one knew any different. Angela in her clinical work outfits cleansed the massage room with the sharp fragrances of essential oils. She was professional, expected her clients on time, plied the tension out of their bodies, and listened to their cares. Women of all ages took to her warm discipline.

Arun was the king of the school. Regular clients as well as those who had just walked off the street listened to him and were drawn to his authentic Himalayan teaching. He attracted private clients and taught them his advanced course for five thousand euros in cash. These men and women had reached the top echelons of their fields—medicine, law, business—but wanted something more: to partake of his peace and well-being. Some became instructors themselves and worked with us or went on to open their own centers in the city.

I maintained my role of administrator, standing faithfully by Arun, but Angela told me I was too quiet, I needed to speak more with the clients. So when they lingered at the desk before class, I asked questions and retained small details about their lives. Soon I knew who had an ailing parent and who was overworked, and I followed up on their next visit. If they were there to complain about their expired class cards, I kept a positive mindset and found a solution. Getting to know our clients—listening and responding to their experiences—became my favorite part of owning the school.

City Yoga was both a business and our home, and on days when I didn't have to go into my corporate office, I attended Arun's early morning class, then drank coffee and ate pastries with Angela and him. One morning, while we were still sipping our drinks, he suddenly left his seat and marched to the entrance. I asked him where he was going, but he ignored me. His silent determination unnerved me, and I followed him out and renewed my question, but he still refused to answer. I insisted, holding his arm, and Angela, who had been watching us, rushed to our side and tried to mediate.

I stared her down. "Don't you ever interfere when a wife is speaking to her husband."

She pouted and walked away.

Arun returned to the reception area and plopped down on the bench. "Never mind."

I couldn't make sense of his furtive behavior. "What is it? Where were you going?"

He looked at me. "There are things I can't tell you. The way you pressed me it won't work anyway."

Angela glared, and I narrowed my eyes at her. She got up and went to the massage room. Finally, I could speak to my husband without the weight of her gaze.

"I was going to play Lotto, and we would have won. But I couldn't tell anyone what I was doing."

Lotto? Was that all? Since our return to Paris, he had picked up what I assumed from his US case files was an old habit. He played the same number of tickets each week—seventy euros' worth. It seemed like a huge amount to gamble for such a slim chance, but he was adamant about not breaking the streak, and if he was ever away, he instructed me to play on his behalf. I didn't think we would win anything significant, but who was I to question his faith?

"This was the one. It would have settled us for life. Now the chance is gone. It won't come again for a long time." His eyes looked dimmed.

He sounded so sure, but I struggled to believe I had the power to break his luck.

On Saturday, I asked Tao about the incident before Angela arrived. The food was ready in the kitchen, and we sat on the floor by the window.

As usual, he sounded more reasonable than Arun. "Someday he will win. I can't tell you when, but he will. When that happens, the money will come to you. I'm working on it for you."

He shook his head. "He doesn't know how to hang on to money. You will be in control of it. I only ask one thing from you: that you take care of both of them."

His face looked hopeful and innocent. "Remember, you and I stand together. Blood is thicker than water." My brother. Beyond Arun and Angela.

Since Angela had come into our life, Tao did the drinking, or at least I assumed he did as Arun abstained. When he and I were alone, we rediscovered our closeness and intimacy—as if the two of us were a team against them. He put up with Angela out of duty to his best friend, who was also an elder on the other side, but he loved me only and wished it were otherwise. He apologized to me in advance in case he ever hugged her out of unconscious habit, and though I didn't comment, I knew I wouldn't be able to handle it. It was hard enough to accept our three-way friendship.

He tried to speak with me about Tao and Angela's sex life, but I wanted to hear nothing of it. Whatever they did together belonged to them; it was no concern of mine.

One day, when the three of us were together, he said to Angela, "You know more about sex than most women."

She looked at him in silence.

I could never quite tell how she saw our strange bond. She seemed happy enough, though her moods fluctuated rapidly from light to dark, and on some level, I didn't consider her feelings. She had entered our lives: I hadn't invited her in.

WHEN ARUN WENT to India at the start of the summer, I looked forward to spending time alone with her. We would finally have a chance to speak unencumbered, and I expected our conversations to expand naturally. I invited her over for a meal on a Friday evening and chose the Italian food she liked but Arun didn't eat. While I prepared the appetizers, I started to chat while she sat on the bed. Her answers were brief, and she seemed reticent to engage. I assumed she might be tired and would perk up over the meal, but when she remained glum, I asked what the matter was.

She sighed. "I just miss them, that's all."

So soon after Tao and Arun had gone? I liked the break from Arun and hadn't started missing him. I tried to make light of the situation. "They'll be back soon. Let's enjoy this time together."

She shrugged. "Yeah."

Her mood sat heavily between us. Her mind was elsewhere, and the pleasant evening I had imagined with my closest friend became a strained effort. She left soon after the meal, and with her departure, my sense of dread lifted. I breathed more easily, cleared up the dishes, and put on an episode of *Friends*.

She showed a cheerful face to Arun and our clients. Why had she been so pensive when we were alone together? I didn't renew my invitation, and she made none of her own.

When Arun returned, she resumed her animated interactions. Over lunch one day, she put down her napkin and exclaimed, "Joelle is the prettiest, most feminine woman I have ever met."

It was an obvious exaggeration, but I was touched by her exuberance—though I did find her choice of words peculiar. I didn't see myself as "pretty" or "feminine." Pretty evoked pink bows and frilly dresses in my mind, and how could I be feminine when I shunned what society considered feminine? I didn't wear skirts or heels, and preferred cotton underwear to the lace thongs she liked. Surely she was the feminine one, not me. No matter how hard I tried I would never understand her.

When Saby visited Dad over the summer, she came to City Yoga and met Angela. Later she told me, "She looks like you. A straight-haired version of you."

It hadn't occurred to me that there was any similarity between us, but Saby had the ability to cut straight to the heart of the matter. She must have picked up on a deeper connection. She returned another time and chatted with Angela. They got along, and we made plans to go see a movie together. In the darkness of the theater, Angela took my hand in a gesture of close friendship. I worried about how it would look to Saby but didn't want to forcibly extract my hand. When she caught a glance of our interlaced fingers, she looked away immediately. She left quickly after the film and didn't suggest another outing. She hardly ever mentioned Angela again after that.

When Mom came to see me later that summer, she visited City Yoga and was impressed by our clientele. I introduced her to a few of our regular clients, and she said, "I would go for coffee with any of them."

Angela greeted Mom with an enthusiastic welcome and kissed her on both cheeks. She was at her best in front of other people when she could be open and radiate her Mediterranean warmth. Mom liked her and later asked me how we had found her. I told her about Gabriel's introduction, and she concluded, "You have a good team."

City Yoga presented well: Gabriel and Angela, two attractive young people, flanked our Indian guru; a spacious locale at a prestigious address; manners, decorum, yoga classes, and a massage offering. Mom could almost set aside her deep dislike of Arun.

Angela, in particular, made an impression on her. "I wouldn't call her beautiful, but she's attractive."

Angular features, striking grey eyes, a petite compact frame. I knew what she meant but didn't want her to analyze Angela. "She looks fine."

"Well, I'm happy for you. She seems to like you a lot."

If only our friendship could be as simple as it seemed.

On his return from India, Arun turned his attention to Angela's professional future. He said her massage training wasn't enough; she needed a degree. She had planned to enroll in a physiotherapy program in Portugal, and he encouraged her to apply to relevant universities in Paris.

He'd spoken to her at our apartment, and after she left, we sat facing each other by the window. He looked at me with a satisfied smile. "Can you imagine her sitting in her own office waiting for patients?"

She seemed so young, insecure, and difficult. "No, I can't."

"She will someday, you'll see."

I resented the note of pride in his voice, the promising future he saw for her. I gazed at the buildings across the street for a moment, then returned to him. "She'll leave us."

His eyes were still illuminated. "She won't."

Buses and cars roared past on the avenue.

"She'll want something more someday."

"We'll see."

"It has to happen," I insisted. Could he not see it? A successful professional wouldn't want to remain in a triad in which she could never introduce her partner. Arun was right to encourage her development, but didn't he see it would end our relationship?

I was deeply divided about the place she had taken in our lives and what her departure would mean. She was an integral part of the school—one leg of the four-legged stool we formed with Gabriel—and she calmed Arun's volatility. I couldn't imagine the school without her, yet I so wished our ties ended there. I longed for the time before she became Tao's wife, the innocence before our complicated bonds.

I wanted Arun to reassure me we would always be enough for each other; we would never need anyone else.

As if reading my thoughts, his expression turned serious. "Jo, if you want me to end this, you need to tell me. I can make sure Tao never comes back."

The summer breeze blew the curtains from the window. I shifted in my seat. "How?'

His eyes turned dark. "I have my ways. I still have power on the other side. Since I killed that elder, they know I can do it."

"No, I don't want that."

"I'm just telling you. You are the one holding this together. The day you don't want it, it will end."

I let out a long exhale. How could I ask Arun to kill my brother?

22

PAST LIVES

Angela applied to two universities. When she received a rejection letter from one, Arun asked me to enlist Dad's help. Dad put me in contact with someone he knew in the system, and within days of my conversation with this man, the second university sent her a positive response. She was elated with the news, and I shared in her joy. She deserved to progress in life.

Arun told her about her illustrious past as the daughter of Gourd Immortal or Hulu Weng. Her closest friend in Portugal was of Chinese descent, and she could see now why she had been drawn to her. Tao and her enlightened parentage, along with Arun and me, completed her new family. Udo, the child-like spirit who had never had a body, recognized her, and she met his attention with reciprocal affection. As both the daughter and the wife of an elder, she was an extraordinary person.

Arun detected signs of our exceptional destinies in our fingerprints. "If you look carefully, Angela's are all closed circles. Yours are all open. That's very rare."

We held our palms open, searching for the patterns.

He looked at us knowingly. "It's extremely powerful to meet two women with such rare, opposite prints."

Did that mean we would win the Lotto? Although I resented any suggestion that Angela and I were on equal footing, angles in the same triangle base, I sensed our shared destiny. She was smart, hardworking, determined, and intense; the only other person who knew about and understood Arun's spirit-channeling and travels to the other side.

I examined my fingers. It was hard to see the rings; maybe they were all open. Maybe Arun was right and there was something special about the two of us. I just hoped the reward would justify the pain of our triad.

By the start of our second year at the school, Gabriel invited us to his studio apartment to meet his new girlfriend. Of Chinese descent, she was a tall, soft-spoken woman with an open oval face. Angela took to her straightaway. They exchanged phone numbers and made plans to see each other again.

Later when we were alone, Arun revealed that she had been Angela's sister in a past life. He had already shared with me his theory of reincarnation, in which only a soul in a healthy body returns intact to their next life. A soul dying in a sick body splits in the afterlife, and returns, weakened, in three or five different bodies. His theory of the increasing number of soul fragments explained not only population growth but why human beings had become less intelligent and more brutish. Angela had recognized her sister in Gabriel's girlfriend and was naturally drawn to her. Then he added that Tao had been married to both sisters in his past life.

I didn't care. He might have had multiple wives in the past, but polygamy was illegal, and he couldn't repeat the practice.

Next Arun identified Silvia, one of our regular clients, as another fragment of Angela's sister's soul. She was charming and gregarious and had attended our classes almost from the opening. She was exceptionally supple and followed instructions with calm attention and a radiant smile. She became Angela's massage client and befriended the two of us. With this second identification of a sister, I wondered if Arun was hinting that Tao wanted to gather his former wives. It was untenable, and I made a point of shutting down the possibility. "He can only have one wife this time."

When Gabriel broke up with his girlfriend, Arun dropped the subject of Angela's sisters.

That autumn he taught me a new practice while we sat in the matted hall for an early practice before any clients arrived. He occupied the teacher's place, and I faced him to his right. He asked me to silently repeat an incantation, "I will not die, I will leave my body," in time with my breaths. I dropped my head and started. The words felt familiar; leaving my body at will was an experience I had fathomed but rejected in fear. If Arun was teaching it to me now, I must be ready. When the time came, my soul would leave as one unit.

Once when Angela and I were at home together after she had been with us a few months, I tried to tell her about my past with Arun, fill in details she had missed, particularly where and how we met, and the drastic change he underwent in Europe. Since she had known him in her past life and felt close to us now, she might help me understand; together we might piece together his mystery. As I started to speak, she cut me off. "I don't want to know about the past."

Her abrupt response to my attempt to open up shocked me. I had known Arun for more than eight years by then. What did she think—that our life together only started when she walked into City Yoga? Didn't she worry that what she didn't know could hurt her? How could she be so sure of her position in our world? We had moments of closeness when she lent me one of her CDs and we listened together, but her unwillingness to hear my story hurt me more than her love of Tao. She couldn't help wanting to be with her former husband, but she had a choice to listen to me.

Her refusal tugged at the knot in my belly. How could we have been so close in a past life yet be so distant now? I searched my mind for memories from that time but couldn't find anything specific. Nothing other than the vision that had appeared to me once in meditation: I had died in her arms. Perhaps I died first last time, leaving Arun and her in pain. Was that why she both loved and pushed me away now?

I voiced my question to Arun. "Did Angela and I really know each other in a past life?"

He looked at me with attention. "Yes, why do you ask?"

"She seems so different this time around."

"She was born in Portugal. You grew up in New York. You've had different life experiences. That's all."

That wasn't it. I searched for words to express what I felt but couldn't find any.

THAT AUGUST, in the middle of our second year, we were able to close the school for a couple of weeks, and our team traveled to Rishikesh. I booked and paid for Angela's ticket, and Gabriel arranged his own travel. The trip would be a journey to Arun's origins. Gabriel and Angela had never been to northern India, and she sensed the country held clues to her past lives.

On our first morning there, I walked out to the veranda and inhaled the scent of earth after the rain. Two years since my last visit and so much had happened. We had partnered with Gabriel, founded our own business, attracted clients, and developed the massage offering with Angela. From nothing, we had responsibilities, and though it had been my dream—and still was—I bore the weight of our financial commitments. Here in the hills, I could enjoy a meditative pause.

I returned inside and found Angela making coffee in the

kitchen. I asked her how she had slept, and she scrunched her face. "It was very noisy outside my room. Till late in the night."

"Oh. I didn't hear anything."

"Your room doesn't face the road."

I opened my mouth, but no words came out.

As she finished pouring the filter coffee into her cup, I reached for the pot, but she held on to it and poured the contents into a second cup. "I'll drink it later."

I didn't see the point of saving coffee which would soon cool but knew better than to argue. As she walked away, I asked, "Do you want to practice together a bit later? Up on the roof? The view is amazing."

She looked withdrawn. "No, I'm going to take it slow today."

She went to her room and closed the door behind her.

I brought out cups of coffee for Arun and me on the veranda. A trace of coolness lingered in the air.

"Where's Angela?" he asked.

"In her room." My gaze settled on the potted plants lining the external wall.

"She doesn't want to come out and enjoy this?"

"She seems tired."

Did he miss her presence? It troubled me that he might— even when the two of us had a quiet moment together.

"How will Tao visit here?" I asked.

Teju, the servant Arun had hired to look after the house, lived in a room adjoining the main building. He had relatively little to do in our absence, but when Arun visited, he cooked, cleaned, and attended to him. Apart from his mid-afternoon break, he came in to make breakfast and left only in the evening.

"Tao will come later, leave earlier."

"He'll sleep in the guest room?"

He watched for my expression. "Yes. Unless you want to give him your room."

In the final house decorations, he had asked Angela to pick the color of the guest room walls since she would be sleeping there. She wanted purple, and her room was painted a deep amethyst shade. I wouldn't give up the air-conditioning and sleep on the other side of the house in that dark hue, surrounded by Angela's energy.

"No, I don't want to leave my room."

Gabriel stayed at a neighboring ashram where Arun had arranged a room for him. He was amazed by the view of the Ganges and fell into the rhythm of life in Rishikesh. Sheltered from Angela's moods and our complicated relationship, he arrived in the morning, sometimes early enough to eat a cooked breakfast of hot cereal or eggs with chilis and wheat flatbreads, then joined us for a walk along the river.

We walked toward Muni Ki Reti, the tourist area, and stopped at the Ganges Guest House, where Arun and I had met. I guided Gabriel and Angela through the unlit reception area and peeked through the closed gift shop. The lingering scent of sweet incense permeated the place. I remembered my first striking vision of Arun sitting self-absorbed in a plastic chair—the ordinary afternoon unexpectedly full of potential—and showed them where we used to chat in the evenings. None of us would be together now if I hadn't met him then, brought him out of India, married him in France, and encouraged him to pursue his calling as a yoga teacher. Gabriel followed my tour with a gentle smile, but Angela moved quickly to the exit, as if she didn't want to absorb my memories.

Her lack of curiosity about the couple whose life she shared so intimately astounded me. Did she never wonder how an American woman in her early twenties met an Indian yogi in his mid-fifties? There was no Tao without Arun and me—did she not realize that? Her taciturn indifference irritated me.

By nine, heat already rose from the earth in a cloying vapor. We continued our walk to the suspension bridge across the wide grey-green expanse of the Ganges, and inched through the press of people and orange-clad swamis shaking the coins in their brass begging bowls. Monkeys scaled the bridge wires, observing us from above.

On the opposite bank, the crowd spread out among street carts. Music blared from the CD seller, as the penetrating sharpness of incense blended with the smell of fried snacks. I took our group to my favorite place—the bookshops—a bit further down the bank, away from the main bustle. In the air-conditioned sanctum, I inhaled the smell of old paper and ink. The bookseller remained silent behind the counter and left us free to explore the shelves. I was always on the lookout for new titles to elucidate the mysteries of the secret practice, and picked up any that spoke of an inner fire and awakening dormant energy.

By the time we retraced our steps up the river, heat permeated the atmosphere. We stopped at a boulder beach, and I removed my shoes and went to dip my feet in the icy water. Angela looked on with concern and called out. "You'll catch an infection."

I yelled back, "No, I won't." A moment later I walked back and showed her my soles, pink and intact.

Before heading home, we stopped at a cafe overlooking the roaring river. Angela ordered tea while the rest of us chose cool drinks. The view of the river and the hills was breathtaking, but my skin itched with prickly heat. I went to the bathroom to splash cold water on my face, but as soon as I returned to the table, I felt the trickle of perspiration down my back and the flush in my cheeks. When we finished our drinks, I said, "I think I need to go."

Angela looked at me in alarm. "Already? But it's so beautiful here."

"I can't cool down. I need to take a shower." We still needed to walk more than half an hour to get home, and I needed to motivate myself.

The men didn't mind. Gabriel would join the tourists who gathered at the local carpenter's house near his ashram. He not only fashioned our bamboo exercise poles but had also learned to carve Aboriginal didgeridoos. He catered to the foreign crowd that met outside his workshop to play music and socialize.

Angela wasn't pleased, but she got up with a pout and followed behind us.

In our second and last week there, she developed an intestinal illness. Her clear skin turned sallow, and her straight back curved. After a couple of days with no improvement, Surat, who was still Arun's local general manager, brought a doctor to see her at home. He gave her an injection, and when he left, I went to check on her in her room. She lay on the bed propped up on pillows, her eyes lined with dark shadows. She appeared listless and looked unfocused. A half-drunk glass of salted lime water was left on her bedside table beside open cosmetic bottles.

I sat by her side and told her I was worried.

"Don't be. I'll be fine."

"Are you taking your dehydration tablets?"

She nodded slowly and stared out the window.

I waited for a moment. "Do you miss Tao?"

The fan whirled at low speed in the still afternoon air.

"Sometimes I feel him around me. But usually he's too far, I can't reach him." Before I could think of a response, she turned and looked at me. "I knew what I was getting into, you know."

I held her gaze for a moment, then looked away. I didn't know what else to say and left her room.

I walked out to the patio where raindrops darkened the tiles and parted the veil of humidity. Plants absorbed the water, and a fresh scent filled the air. I breathed it all in. I couldn't fix the situation for Tao and Angela. All I could do was watch and hope one day there would be a solution.

On our last evening in Rishikesh, Arun said to me, "Surat asked about her."

"Oh yeah? What did he say?"

"He said, 'I don't know what your relationship is to that woman, but I can see you're close.'"

The knot in my belly tightened. "What did you tell him?"

He looked at me in the semi-darkness.

"I said, 'We're close, that's all.'"

That wasn't the right answer. He should have said, "There is nothing between us."

I didn't know what he expected from me, but he had to protect the sanctity of our marriage. That was all I asked of him.

23

SACRIFICE

Arun and I had discussed sharing City Yoga's profits with Gabriel and Angela, but without consulting with me he gave them each a one-page document granting them twenty percent of the profits. In a way, it didn't matter: if he had asked me, I would have agreed. The school was our family business, each of us a leg in its foundation. And profit was still a long way off. Our clientele had grown, but the cost of renting a commercial unit in central Paris, along with teachers' wages, outstripped our revenues. Our initial investment of close to a hundred thousand euros needed to be repaid. I hadn't expected riches from the school, but I had hoped to earn enough to be able to leave my corporate job. I had been working in Paris, managing my UK team remotely, for close to three years, and while being in charge of the sales commission process was considered an important role, I knew my job inside out and could breeze through the day.

After the trip to Rishikesh, I turned my attention to City Yoga's finances and hired an accountant. We were late in filing our taxes and had months of entries to update in the bookkeeping software. The task was monumental, and I solicited the team to split it up among us. Gabriel agreed to take on a portion, but Angela declined. Accounting wasn't her area of expertise, and she didn't have time now that she had started her university course. At a moment when we needed to pull together, her explanation made me bristle. Arun tried to help but made so many errors that I took over his share.

Our accountant, Alex, was a soft-spoken African-French man with round metal glasses. A few weeks after we handed over the accounts to him, he returned with a satchel full of documents. His message was unfiltered: the business didn't make enough money to support us. If we wanted to live from the school, we would have to open a few more establishments across the city.

His assessment disheartened me, and I sought Arun's counsel. "When do you think I'll be able to leave my job?"

"Why do you want to leave?"

"It's not my calling. I want to work full-time at the school."

"The company needs you. They won't find a more honest worker."

"But do you think they'll let me go eventually? I've been a senior manager for years, and I'm not developing my career."

"They won't let you go. You do important work there."

His vision might not reflect my wish, but I trusted his instincts and accepted his pronouncement.

Since we opened the school, I had been having a recurring dream. I was at the desk managing reception, but it was a different place, much vaster than our yoga hall: a large, open, thatched hut on a tropical island. Gabriel was teaching, and so many students arrived at once to attend his class that I couldn't keep track of who had signed in or who had paid. In the end, I gave up: the register couldn't contain the number of people in the hall. Although the dream was fraught with anxiety—over my inability to stay on top of the crowd and the finances—I was also swept away by abundance: we were so successful that I had lost control.

While Angela balanced her university studies with her client load, Gabriel had started to teach yoga at other establishments in the city. He had even come to the attention of famous yoga gurus in New York City and was invited to give a workshop at their studio there. He relished the effect of his impressive performance and personal magnetism; his yoga stardom was on the rise. For me, though he had just turned twenty-nine, he hadn't changed from the charming young man I had met three years earlier. We didn't speak much, but when he passed by me at reception on his way to teach, he smiled in his familiar gentle manner.

One morning, when the temperature had dropped and the day was still dark, I arrived at the school, booted the computer, and found a pile of pages on the printer. I picked them up and saw that each sheet had incomplete client data. Some showed their emails, others their names and phone numbers. Strange. Someone had obviously tried to print off the client list but hadn't managed to fit all the data on one sheet. Our client file, apart from being confidential, was our most valuable asset. Only one person had been at the school after we closed the evening before.

I put in a call to the cleaner who came in after the classes were done and asked if she had seen Gabriel at the computer during her shift. She was reluctant to answer me at first, but after I reassured her that I needed the information and no harm would come from it, she said that he had been at the computer when she arrived but was gone by the time she had finished cleaning the hall. I was shocked by her confirmation and asked Arun if he thought Gabriel might have tried to steal our client data.

"If he did, he won't ever step in here again. I don't care what excuse he gives."

It was hard to imagine Gabriel, who knew the pain of our start-up and our difficulty in turning a profit, operating on his own and working against us. City Yoga might not offer the same glamour as some of the other places where he was asked to teach, but he was family.

That evening, I joined Arun at reception. As usual, Gabriel whisked in a few minutes before his class, a backpack slung on one shoulder, and met us with a quick smile before rushing to the men's changing room.

Arun stopped him in his tracks. "I need to speak with you."

"My class is starting in a few minutes."

Arun held up the stack of papers. "What's this?"

Gabriel blinked and looked away, but before Arun could say anything else, students walked through the door. He turned his attention to them, and Gabriel went in to prepare.

After the class started, I asked what Arun planned to do.

"I'm going to kick him out."

"Who will teach tomorrow?"

"I will."

"In the evening?"

He moved his head from side to side in confirmation. "If he thinks he can put a leg over me, he's wrong."

I rested my elbows on the table and rubbed my temples. Despite the enormity of Gabriel's betrayal, I didn't look forward to his departure, even if it felt like he had already left.

When the class ended and all the students were gone, Arun confronted him again.

Gabriel looked down. "I wanted to send an email about my workshop. That's all."

Arun had already packed his belongings in a plastic bag and handed it to him. "Here's your stuff."

Gabriel looked at him with glistening eyes and apologized, but it was too late.

"Get out of my sight. You tried to hurt us. I don't like traitors."

Gabriel hoisted his backpack on one shoulder, took the plastic bag in the other hand, and marched into the night. He didn't turn back or say goodbye.

WE SOON FILLED the gap he left in the schedule with other teachers, and even his most faithful clients accepted the change. A few asked where he'd gone, and when I answered that he had moved on, they didn't say anything more.

But what I couldn't replace was his presence in our lives. He was Arun's first friend in Europe, close to both of us before we had the school. Without him, we wouldn't have taken the step of founding City Yoga. In my dream of overflowing students, he was always at the helm, and though the vision would return in the years ahead, it no longer felt like a positive prophecy.

Mostly I missed his carefree presence. How he made our triangle into a square: the base of the school, the foundation of something normal. I doubted he knew about Angela's closeness to us, but if he was sensitive, he might have realized that Arun treated her differently. Did he feel slighted? I didn't think so. He was simply swept on his own trajectory to stardom, amazed and gratified by his effect on others and their validation of his worth. I missed the time before Angela, when everything was still possible.

Given their earlier friendship, she said surprisingly little about his departure. She followed Arun's lead, and maybe on her new path Gabriel wasn't so important anymore. This was what I assumed. She didn't share her feelings with me, nor did I with her. Perhaps she had other concerns.

Since her bout of illness in Rishikesh, her appearance had

changed considerably. Her strong, compact body had hollowed out, her bright eyes filled with shadows. I couldn't help expressing concern about her weight loss, but she was quick to answer me. "You didn't know me when I lived in Portugal. I was always like this. I only gained weight in Paris after I lost my job."

"Well, be careful not to lose too much."

"Don't worry. I feel much better now."

Her happy insouciance didn't convince me.

I also noticed the change in her eating habits over Saturday lunch. She picked at her food and left clumps of rice on her plate.

"Don't you like it?" I asked.

"I can't eat so much." She patted her stomach. "I'm so full."

Another time, she said the food was too greasy, so I asked what she liked.

"It's fine. Don't change anything for me."

Arun didn't comment on the change in her, and I wondered what was going on.

One day she announced out of the blue with satisfaction on her face, "If I ever get married, it'll be to a woman."

Her comment didn't surprise me. She had accepted to be the lover of a ghost who was mostly absent. What kind of life did she have with him? Maybe she didn't want to spend that much time with a man and envisioned a future with a woman.

When months passed with no sign of recovery, I asked Arun what he thought might be troubling her. We were sitting on the floor having our first cup of coffee by the window. I woke up fresh with ideas, and we often conferred and discussed matters at this time.

He appeared surprised. "What do you mean?"

"She's so thin. I don't think she enjoys eating with us anymore."

"She might be worried about her studies."

That wasn't it. "Do you think she might be anorexic?"

"I don't think so. Why are you so worried all of a sudden?"

I searched my mind. "Maybe she doesn't want to be with us anymore."

"Don't say that. She loves us."

"You maybe, but not me. She's only here for Tao."

"That's not true. She looks up to you."

"But she hardly talks to me."

There were still times when we relaxed together, listening to music or watching a show; but too often, I sensed her pain. Even if Arun refused to admit it, something had changed since Rishikesh. I dropped the topic but picked it up again when Tao visited on Saturday.

As usual, he was more responsive to my concerns. "Being with me takes a lot out of her."

I wanted to ask him: Does it have to be like this? Will you ever have your own body? But as soon as the thought formed in my mind, I realized it made no sense. How would we recognize Tao if he showed up at our door in an unknown body?

No. There would only ever be one body: Arun's.

Tao drew me from my thoughts. "The elders are very proud of you, you know. Very few women in your place would accept this situation."

I was glad he acknowledged how difficult it was for me and hoped my sacrifice would resonate on the other side. I also needed confirmation that I was still Arun's most faithful and worthy student.

"I'm very grateful to you," Tao added.

I was always looking for reassurance, but sometimes his words unsettled me, like the time he looked at me intently and said, "The service she does for us you could never do. But she will never be you. Not in a thousand lifetimes."

What kind of service did he mean? Was she giving up her

life energy to him? And what was my role? What was so different about me?

The knot in my belly would break open someday. But until then, I sacrificed my will for the elders' grace. No matter what Tao said: deep inside, I wanted her gone.

24

BACK TO THE CAVE

By the autumn of 2005, we had been living in Dad's studio for almost four years. What was meant to be a temporary arrangement was dragging on too long. Dad didn't need the apartment for himself but liked to have a place for his guests, so several months after Angela came into our lives, we had given him the use of our studio and found another one for Angela in the building where we lived. She was closer to Tao when he visited, and I found it comforting to know he wasn't far.

We had also started to pay rent after seeing a sign in the building's reception hall about the sale of Dad's studio by auction. We learned the local government was taking control following mounting unpaid property taxes. Arun didn't want to move, and we offered Dad to sign a formal lease with us which would prevent the forced seizure of the property. Once I showed the rental agreement to the tax authorities, they requisitioned the rent. Since I still hadn't been able to return Dad's startup loan for City Yoga, the agreement would allow me to pay him back indirectly over time.

The building had once been a hotel, and all the apartments

were studios. There was something anonymous about it that I found off-putting, but Arun liked. When two apartments, one directly above the other, went up for sale, he suggested that we buy the pair and live in both of them. Angela would then move into Dad's studio.

I didn't like the idea. Not only were the two studios oddly shaped, but I didn't want to live across two properties. I was inspired then and there to consult the real estate section of a major newspaper to see what else might be available, and found a listing that caught my attention: a penthouse close to where we lived and to the school, at a bargain price. It hadn't been touched since the fifties and needed a complete refurbishment, but after viewing it, I was convinced it was the right choice for our permanent home.

Arun continued to push the idea of the studios, which he thought would be a better investment, but I resisted. He had called the financial shots since we met ten years earlier. The very first loan I had given him of thirty thousand dollars was for a good investment in India. He had sworn by Baba he would someday pay me back, but I never heard about the money—or the business—again. In Valbonne, he had invested in penny stocks, sure he would turn a profit, and lost all the money. In Maidenhead, he had convinced me to cash in Nortel options and buy company stock, then the shares plummeted. I didn't regret these misplaced risks or expect him to pay back my initial loan—so much had changed since then. With his encouragement I had pursued an MBA and now had a well-paying job. He had pushed me through those early years when I doubted myself. We had a yoga school together and a retirement property in India. We were a team, he and I. We had taken on projects and accomplished things. I might be more cautious than he was, but I was also more circumspect. The yin to his yang.

But now at the age of thirty-two, I wanted a home of my own.

He pointed out that we would be further from Angela, and that sealed the deal for me. "We can't live our whole life tied to her."

My first bank in Fontainebleau was only too happy for me to sell my two-bedroom apartment, which was still rented to support the loan repayments on our Indian property, and buy one of lesser value. They offered us a bridge loan to secure the purchase until my apartment sold. I bought the new place in our joint names, and the bank encouraged me to borrow more than we needed for the renovations. Our account was flush with cash.

Not missing a chance to convert cash to gold, Arun went to a jewelry sale at an auction house. He returned with a solid gold Rolex watch for himself, an item he had wanted for years, and a diamond solitaire ring and matching gold necklace for me. He even bought a designer steel watch for Angela. Swept up by his enthusiasm for what he considered bargains, I joined him for the Christmas sale, and we made the winning bid for a massive yellow sapphire ring below its listed valuation. Another investment.

We closed on the new apartment at the end of the year, and Arun insisted on hiring the same Pakistani builder who had worked at City Yoga even after I had found a reputable plumbing and electricity company to do the tricky renovation. He wanted the man he knew to take the whole job, despite the trouble he'd caused us at the school. He wanted to be able to boss him around in his native tongue. I had doubts about the decision, but as he would be overseeing the work, I relented. I had enough on my plate with my corporate role and managing the school on the side.

The builder got through the initial stage of breaking down some partition walls, but after that, the work progressed with alarming errors. No matter how much Arun shouted in Urdu over the phone, we had three different plumbers and two major leaks that caused water to flow into the downstairs neighbors' property. The second one took place on a Sunday toward the end of the renovation. The neighbors didn't know how to reach us and called the fire department to break in and cut the water flow. By then the brand-new hardwood floorboards in the living room had been flooded. When we moved in a few weeks later, they were already swollen out of shape. We had spent a huge amount of money—over a hundred thousand euros—on shoddy work. In the final days when there were only a few items to finish, the builder stopped answering his phone. He resurfaced a couple of days later and told Arun he had been in jail.

We moved in at the start of April, after what felt like three interminable months. Arun had chosen a different paint color for each room: salmon-orange for the spacious living room; peppermint ice cream green for the dining room; and cotton candy pink for the bedroom. Jarringly vivid shades, but a minor consequence of leaving him in charge of the renovation. At least the pain of the build was behind us, and we could settle down in our own home now.

Two weeks later, he decided to travel to his cave in the high Himalayas. The timing surprised me—in early spring the roads might still be blocked by snow—but he insisted that he had to go then. I had misgivings about his sudden need to travel so soon after we had moved into the new apartment, but assumed he was responding to a call from the elders and needed to connect with them through the cave's portal—a hidden place where the boundary between the material and spiritual worlds was permeable. He could accomplish work there that he couldn't do in Paris. I accepted his decision and turned my attention to the additional responsibilities I would need to manage without him at the school.

He said to me before leaving, "You give me so much freedom, Jo. You always let me do what I want."

I was proud that he recognized and appreciated the lifestyle I made possible, relieved that my clinging love didn't stifle him.

In his absence, I relished my quiet morning routine: sitting on the handwoven Tibetan carpet, inhaling the penetrating scent of incense, holding my breath while drawing the energy up, then exhaling fully. Breathing in this controlled way led me to a deep space within myself, centered and open. Sometimes when my mind slipped into oblivion, I sensed a gap, and when I opened my eyes, I jotted down thoughts in my journal.

We had a young client at the school, an attractive professional singer with a soft pliable body. Arun liked her, and so did I—even when he implied that she was drawn to us, saying, "if we asked her to move in with us, she wouldn't hesitate." He made prophetic pronouncements about many different people, and this one rang as just one more.

But a week after he left, I awoke in the middle of the night from a nightmare featuring this client. In the dream, he had avoided a relationship with her at first, then changed course and said I had already lost him and he would marry her. I went back to sleep, and he appeared again. This time he told me Angela had another man in her future. To which I answered, "What about me? I don't want anybody else."

I awoke in tears on Sunday morning, full of foreboding.

The following day, the ringing phone interrupted my meditation. It could only be Arun this early in the morning, and I bounded from my seat to answer. His voice croaked over the static on the line. "It's me. Something happened."

"What is it? Where are you calling from?"

"I'm in Uttarkashi. I had an accident."

Uttarkashi was the last town on the way up to Gangotri, the village higher up in the mountains where he had his cave. He wasn't due back for another week. I sat down and clutched the receiver. "What happened?"

The story sounded simple enough: the cave had been very cold, he and Teju had lit a fire to keep warm, and they woke up to smoke. The cave had been constructed in a convenient space between rocks, with a cement structure and a couple of windows.

"Oh my God, did you not open any windows?"

"No, it was very cold."

"Have you been to a doctor?"

"I will. As soon as I get to Rishikesh. I'll call you from there."

The line crackled, and I feared our conversation would be cut. "Arun, I love you."

"I love you too."

My belly tightened with worry as I digested the news. He had been able to ring me, that was a good sign at least. I looked up carbon monoxide poisoning online, and my findings were concerning. Only immediate high doses of oxygen could prevent brain damage. With nothing to do but wait, I opened my work emails and started the day at home.

He called again several hours later when he was back in Rishikesh. The line was clearer, but his voice was still strained. "I can't pee. The doctor says there's something wrong with my pancreas."

"Your pancreas? What do you mean your pancreas? Have you been treated for carbon monoxide poisoning?"

"No."

"Why not?"

"I don't know."

"Well, ask about it."

He sounded confused, and I wondered how quickly I could get to Rishikesh. A couple of days at best. But what would I be able to do that doctors couldn't?

I asked about Teju, and Arun said he had no symptoms. Was it a question of age? Teju was a young man, not yet thirty. Voices sounded in the background, and Arun said he had to go, the doctor had arrived.

I rested my forehead in my hands and took a few slow breaths. Something didn't make sense. Had he really lit a fire, then fallen asleep in a cave with no ventilation? Or had he perhaps been absent, in deep meditation?

Next time we spoke he mentioned an operation on his pancreas.

"I haven't peed since I left the cave. No, no, not my pancreas. I mean my prostate."

"Oh, that makes more sense. Have they given you oxygen?"

"No."

"I read online that oxygen has to be administered immediately to avoid long-term damage."

"They didn't give me any."

"Did you explain to the doctor what happened? Does he know you were poisoned?"

"Yes, I think so."

"Do you want me to come there?"

"No, it's okay, I'll be fine. Surat is here. I'll come home soon."

It wasn't easy to leave the school and my job at the drop of a hat, but if it was necessary, I would have found a way. I feared that since the critical window to administer oxygen had passed, my presence wouldn't make a difference anyway.

My vivid nightmares had taken place the night he was poisoned. I prayed for his healing.

ARUN RETURNED on a Sunday morning at the end of April. He had been gone for three weeks but hadn't managed to do whatever critical work had driven him to the cave. When his key turned in the door, I sprang up to greet him. He dropped his bag and took me in his arms without a word. I breathed in his familiar sweet scent.

When he had freshened up and joined me in the living room, I took a good look at him. He sat on the short side of the L-shaped couch, at a diagonal from me, his checked flannel shirt rolled up to his elbows and his hands clasped over his legs. He looked the same as the man who had left: strong and in control. He focused on me from the depth of his storytelling gaze; the glint in his eyes was the living proof of his survival.

"It was a close one."

"Thank God you're here."

"I fought for my life in the cave."

"What happened?" I moved in closer. "Did something happen?"

He repeated the same facts about the unbearable cold, the fire, falling asleep, then waking up disoriented.

"It's very dangerous. You know how dangerous fire can be."

"We were freezing, I didn't think."

One thoughtless mistake . . . or—

"Was there something else that night?"

He shook his head.

I asked about Teju. Arun said he had been further from the fire and hadn't been affected. I was happy for him, but struggled to understand how a yogi trained in longevity practices had suffered more than someone who had never formally exercised or meditated in his life. For three weeks, Arun's body and mind remained intact, and I was grateful that he too had been spared.

ON A QUIET SUNDAY MORNING, after clearing the breakfast dishes, I walked into the living room. Arun had been sitting there only moments before, but it was empty. I checked the small entrance hallway. His shoes were in their usual place, so he couldn't have gone out. I called out to him, though it was obvious he wasn't there, then went to the balcony to look outside. He was standing on the street by the building doors.

I shouted, "What are you doing there?"

He looked up with a sheepish grin, and I ran down the five flights of stairs, opened the door, and found him in his slippers, hands in his pockets.

"I forgot the code."

Back in the apartment, I scolded him. "Don't just go off like that. I was worried sick. What were you doing?"

"Just buying some beers."

I sighed. He shouldn't be drinking again so soon after the accident, but at least he wasn't lost.

"You went in your slippers."

He looked down at his feet as though noticing them for the first time.

After that incident, I wrote the building code on a piece of paper, and hoped he would remember to take it with him whenever he went out. It soon proved unnecessary as he memorized the six-digit sequence. His memory lapse seemed like an isolated case. But there was something about the way he had gone out in slippers—the vulnerability in his gaze when I went to find him—that put me on alert.

Most of his life skills were unchanged. He could still shave, for instance; perform the delicate task of bringing a blade to his neck. I took comfort in his ability to take care of himself.

But in other areas, particularly his speech, he was a different man. He could string together words into sentences and make himself clear, but he showed little interest in casual conversation, one of his former talents. Our morning chats—about the school, the elders, my corporate work, anything really—had sparked our connection. Now he uttered only the words necessary for daily living. The yogi who had wielded his voice as the instrument of his charm now met the world through a gauze of quiet. The change was too noticeable to attribute to a passing mood, but when I mentioned it to him, he said nothing had changed. Suddenly, without warning, we had lost our shared meaning.

25

PRAYER

Since my move out of Dad's apartment and my rent payments to service his tax debt, our relationship had settled into a strained détente. Still, he was my only family in Paris, and I spoke to him about Arun's accident and the resultant changes in his personality. He suggested a consultation with a neurologist at the private American Hospital, and Lena dropped us off at the appointment in her Mercedes convertible. We arrived with plenty of time to spare and waited for our appointment in a pristine, whitewashed room brightened with late spring light. The other patients around us looked older and frailer than Arun, and in that quiet moment, I was filled with hope.

We were soon called in to see the neurologist and sat across his desk. He examined x-rays of Arun's brain and pointed out the dark spots where the frontal cortex had been damaged. He put the slides away and asked what the problem was, as if the images hadn't been clear enough. Arun kept quiet, so I stepped in and explained his recent memory losses and selective mutism (the term I had learned to explain his diminished verbal engagement).

The neurologist asked him a series of factual questions, all of which he was able to answer, then told him to count in increments of three. He did so without a problem. When he had to count back from a hundred in the same increments, he hesitated then started, "Ninety-seven, ninety-four," and continued from there.

Next, he had to draw a cube, and there he fumbled with the pen and drew a bunch of lines culminating in the same point, like a tepee. "I can't seem to get it."

His voice was soft as a child's. I felt his struggle and asked the doctor if he would heal.

"It's impossible to predict how the brain will respond after injury. Some people heal completely, others not at all."

I was disappointed to leave the hospital with such uncertainty and no further clues about Arun's future despite the hefty bill. He didn't express himself, so I couldn't tell what he thought, but I had to believe he would be one of the lucky ones.

Over the coming days he sank deeper into himself, and when he developed urinary incontinence, he showed the first signs of distress. The first time it happened, he looked down at the stain on his trousers with a stricken expression, and we rushed home. His urge to urinate was uncontrollable, and wherever we went, he always needed to be close to a bathroom.

Dad invited us out to lunch—to cheer us up perhaps—and as soon as we were seated, Arun stood up and looked at me. I found the bathroom and guided him there. I returned to the table, and Dad looked at me compassionately. When the food arrived, Arun slurped his soup with mechanical clicks of his spoon against the bowl and hardly spoke with Dad.

By the start of summer, we planned a short beach holiday, as he wasn't well enough to go to India. Before we left, he said, "This has to stop," and true to his word, as suddenly as it had started, the incontinence came to an end. His self-mastery gave me hope that he would heal completely.

The place where his new persona was the most disturbing was at the school. He got into the habit of wearing heavy pilot headphones and playing video games or watching movies on the office computer. Much of the day he had the place to himself, but when students filtered in before class, he remained tethered to the computer and checked them in silently while muffled sounds of battle leaked from the headphones. It was unseemly, and I wanted to tell him to stop, but he had suffered such a personal setback that I left him alone.

Angela wasn't so forgiving. "Turn it down and take it off." She looked at me in exasperation, and when I didn't respond she exclaimed, "I can't work like this," and stormed to the back room.

She was right; his behavior was anti-social. I tried gentle verbal coaxing, but he ignored me. I touched his shoulder to get his attention, and when he took no notice, I tugged at the mouse. Only then did he turn to me in alarm. "What are you doing?"

I kept my voice low. "You can't do that here."

"I'm not bothering anyone."

"It doesn't fit. We're here to teach yoga and give massages, not play games and watch movies."

His fixation on video games came after years of almost no interest (the reactive joystick from Fontainebleau had long been abandoned after minimal use), and as I watched him in self-absorbed silence I felt like the mother of a sullen child.

"Don't you care about the school anymore?"

He slid the mouse across the desk and left his seat.

Months went by with little sign of improvement, and I asked our teachers to be present at reception before their classes. It wasn't technically part of their job, and I'm sure they would have preferred going into the hall to prepare, but they understood my request. They believed in their work and needed their salaries, and Arun's unfriendly behavior wasn't helping to welcome clients, especially those who were discovering the school for the first time.

Angela still came over for lunch on Saturdays, but now that we were in our new home, a ten-minute walk from hers, her visits were shorter. She was eager to return to her studies. Arun's cooking had always been spicier than I would have liked, but after his brain injury he lost all sense of measure, as if his tastebuds had been dulled. Angela nibbled at her food, and I stopped asking about her tastes or worrying about her gaunt state. There was no sense in meddling.

On a rare occasion she lingered after the meal and spoke with me after Arun had gone to watch television. "He's changed so much. How do you cope with it?"

I shrugged. "What can I do about it?"

She gazed outside the window. "Does he speak when the two of you are alone together?"

"Not much."

She sighed. "Tao's the same."

"The other day he started smoking again."

Her grey eyes opened wide.

"For a minute, after he took the first puff, he paid attention to me." I smiled. "It was Tao actually. He asked how my work was going. That hadn't happened in a long time." It had been very pleasant to feel Tao's caring attention after so long—the return of the man I remembered, not the aloof Arun I lived with now.

Her expression remained somber. "I don't think he should be smoking in the state he's in."

There she was, critical again.

"Look, it's part of his life. He's not about to stop now. Plus, it's the one thing he really enjoys."

She looked away again, and I thought she was done, but then she whispered, "It's hard to connect with Tao now."

It was my cue to show empathy, but I didn't feel any. Not for her, who had lodged herself deep inside my marriage as if she belonged there.

"They've had an accident."

"I know."

"So what should we do? Abandon them when they're down?"

"I didn't say that. I would never say that."

Arun had once said to me, while we still lived at Dad's studio, "You will wake up in New York, and Angela will wake up in Porto."

His statement startled me. Wake up? From what? "Why there?"

"You will wake up in your original home."

To wake up implied coming into some previously hidden knowledge. I caught a glimpse of his meaning: perhaps we weren't living our most authentic lives here in Paris—with him and Tao.

"Where will you wake up?" I asked.

He seemed surprised by my question, as if he wasn't in the same category as Angela and me. After a beat, he said, "I'll wake up in Rishikesh."

Perhaps it had been bold to imply that he, too, was asleep; but his assertion suggested a time would come when we would all separate.

By 2007, a year after Arun's accident, four since we opened City Yoga, our business was stagnating. Two years since Gabriel left, we were nowhere near my anxiety-fueled dreams of uncontrolled crowds; we weren't even breaking even.

At the first anniversary of the three-year lease, I had negotiated to keep the rent unchanged and pushed my relationship with the property agent to its limits. He found me difficult and argumentative, but I had obtained a temporary reprieve from our mounting costs. The rent was bound to increase again next year, and I decided to seek business counsel from one of Arun's private clients, a senior venture capital partner who had become a friend.

He came to City Yoga and met with our team: Arun, Angela, and me, as well as a senior yoga instructor I had asked to join us. Arun sat behind the desk, the rest of us on chairs and the teak bench. After opening the meeting, our friend asked us each to suggest ideas for improving the business. When it was Angela's turn, she became defensive: her load was full, and she couldn't do any more. He responded that it wasn't about doing more, but her face was set in a pout and she kept quiet. Arun thought we could raise class fees significantly, but none of us agreed. I don't remember what the other yoga instructor had in mind, but she didn't stay very long, and after she left, our friend contemplated the three of us.

"I've met a lot of management teams, and I can tell you all haven't gelled yet. The management team—how well they work together—is critical to business success."

He meant to encourage us, but he didn't know half our story.

I knew we were doomed.

Amidst business strains and Arun's stagnation, his former wife in Delhi resurfaced. He was now sixty-seven, and I assumed she was of similar age. She couldn't make ends meet, and he asked me to send her a monthly stipend of two hundred euros. Though a small portion of our overall budget, it was one more cost to absorb in my monthly salary. Still, I respected his commitment to his original family, and we couldn't turn away when she had no other means to support herself. I counted the payment as a charitable contribution.

The following year, she needed a cataract operation, and I sent two thousand euros. I had learned from living with Arun to spend nothing on myself and still accepted Mom's regular gifts of clothes. I drew on my savings to cover the unexpected medical expense.

Long ago Arun had mentioned being adopted but never spoke of living parents. When they died within a year of each other, as the eldest son, he returned to India to preside over their funeral rites. His sudden observance of filial duty caught me by surprise. After keeping their existence hidden, he called them Mom and Dad in Hindi. Yet he revealed nothing about them—not even at their deaths—and I didn't pick up any sadness when he received the news of their passing. Arun operated according to his own, often mysterious, principles and rules, and I assumed that as a spirit living in a dead man's body, he was devoid of emotion. After more than a decade together, I still didn't know where he had grown up with his master, Babaji, and learned the secret practice.

Since his accident, I felt bereft: I yearned for the deep connection we once had. Unable to communicate my anguish to him, I wrote in my journal. "That part of me that is hungry for your words, nothing else can fill. We ask even the gods to speak with us, why not you?"

One evening, I sat on the warped wooden floor by my bookcase in the living room. Night had fallen, and Tao had gone to Angela's. A spontaneous prayer formed in my mind. *God, please restore Arun's voice. Even to speak with you, we use words. Please don't abandon me in a world of silence with no end.*

Speaking with God lifted my burden. I knew he would hear me.

PART IV

SEEDS OF LIFE

26

SECOND CHANCE

When Saby invited me to her wedding in New York early in 2009, Arun wanted to attend with me. Although we had learned years earlier that his return would be impossible, I thought his interest might stem from the elders' advice, and we applied for his visa at the US Embassy. I had made many trips to New York since our move to Europe and had accepted that my life would always be split in two: the comfort and safety of Mom's home and the chaos and potential of living with Arun. But if his criminal record had expired, we might be on the verge of a new fate. He didn't lie on his visa application—that would have been too risky—and the negative answer was swift. I wasn't surprised, but the failure felt like one more sign of stagnation.

Two weeks before I would travel on my own, I lay on the living room couch, shivering under a blanket. Arun was lying on the other end in the same condition. It was a Monday afternoon, and I had gone to bed after the sudden onset of flu symptoms when my colleague phoned to tell me the CEO had invited all employees to an impromptu call and I'd want to hear his message. I connected to the call just in time to hear him announcing that Nortel had filed for Chapter II bankruptcy protection.

Three months earlier my manager had summoned our whole department to a meeting in Miami, a combined learning and reward session by the beach. At the end of the conference, she addressed the forty members of our global team and told us of difficult times ahead. We had been working for years without bonuses, and I had made it through multiple rounds of layoffs, but the company was still struggling. We might hear concerning news about the sale of the most lucrative business unit, but she promised to share more information as soon as she could. Despite her calm and measured southern tone, we were worried. But we hadn't anticipated the CEO's message: all four business units would be sold, not just "the crown jewels." My physical state mirrored the company's financial situation.

After the shock of the initial announcement, I watched and waited. My most ambitious colleagues found jobs elsewhere, but I didn't know how to market myself to other companies or what aspect of my role I would want to retain. For the last six years, I had depended on my remote working arrangement with Nortel to devote most of my energy to City Yoga. I had no idea how I would replicate this situation elsewhere—or indeed if I could.

Over the next six months the four business units were sold to different companies, and by summer my analyst team split by affiliation. As the manager, I worked across the business and wasn't assigned to any of the acquiring companies; I would remain employed at the French branch until liquidation, then qualify for the minimum government redundancy payment. It was a huge setback.

On a Saturday afternoon in August, I awoke from a long nap in the living room. Arun had returned from his spirit travels and sat on the other side of the room staring into space. His slim aquiline nose still defined his profile, but his grey hair had thinned down to strands. His muscular structure and strong bones had outlived years of indulgent living, but his belly protruded. He had always spent the afternoons sitting in front of the television, then traveling to the other side, but since his accident he had become more rooted in place, mechanical in his movements. Our space was thick with silence.

I sat up and looked at him, and a realization hit me: all our achievements in Europe had been down to me. Without my job at Nortel, we wouldn't have our long-term French residencies; we wouldn't have obtained multiple mortgage approvals. If it weren't for my salary—working at a job that I might not value but had performed conscientiously for close to eleven years— we wouldn't have been able to open the school, supplement its flagging income time and again, and pay rent to house Angela. Every part of our livelihood, down to the extra cash we sent to Arun's family in India, depended on me and my job. When I would soon be out of work, we wouldn't even have the private medical insurance we relied on to address Arun's ailments.

He might have encouraged me to get the MBA degree, but since then, as he had announced after my graduation, he had contributed almost nothing to our household. The elaborate edifice of our life depended completely on my efforts. I held the power—and had done so all along. This galvanizing insight surged through me.

He was about to turn on the television, but I went to his side.

Clutching the remote control, he turned to me. "What's up?"

"I don't think I'll have a job soon."

"Why do you say that?"

"I'm not assigned to any of the companies."

"They need you."

"Not if there's no salespeople."

'We'll see.' He was restless and stared at the dark screen.

"Wait, I'm not done."

He gripped the remote control and paused.

I asked the question that weighed on my mind. "What about Angela?"

I had his attention now. "What if I have a new job and can't keep up with the school?"

"I'll take care of it."

"It's not that easy. Who'll do all the accounting? And the paperwork?"

"Let's see, Jo. Let that time come."

Then I repeated the words I had said to him before. "Will it always be this way?"

He stared.

"Tao coming through you?"

"Why do you ask?"

I shrugged. "It must be hard for them."

He gave me a vague answer, so I asked, "Will he ever have his own body?"

"He would like to, but it's difficult. It took us a long time to find this one." His expression turned somber. "Tao found it for me."

My eyes opened in alarm. "But it's yours, right? He won't ever take over completely?"

His sorrowful eyes rested on me. "He wouldn't do that. He loves you."

IN SEPTEMBER, one of my colleagues told me she was leaving Nortel. Although we worked in different departments, our jobs intersected, and her loss would be felt. I decided to take a chance and phone her manager, whom I knew well. Fiona was an Irish woman with a quick mind and a vivacious personality. As one of the business leaders who decided on sales compensation issues, we had worked together over the years, and I knew she liked me. When I asked her about applying for the open position in her department, she jumped at the idea, then caught herself and asked for a day to sleep on it. I was glad I'd taken the initiative and felt confident about the outcome.

She came back the next day with a positive response, but as the list of employees transferring to the acquiring company was already closed, she would need to work to get my name added. Still, she was exuberant about the possibility and invited me to a sales planning call with Trevor, her counterpart from the acquiring company. He led the discussions in a deep resonant voice and asked me directly if I would be setting the sales targets for the Nortel associates.

"Yes," I said. I had never set sales targets before, but it was the only answer I could give him.

The promise of the new job lifted me out of my despair.

Arun and I went to Rishikesh over the Christmas break. Once I started at the new company, I wouldn't be able to travel for a while, and my nerves were frayed from months of anxiety about the future. I needed the rest and change of scenery.

Arun had taken more funds from France to build a huge hall, twice the size of the one at City Yoga, on the second floor of the house. From the third floor, the view over the Ganges was even more breathtaking, and the hall proved his commitment to developing a school of Agni Yoga in Rishikesh, the origins of the practice he taught in Paris. In a burst of creativity, he had also invented a new series of forward-bending stretches performed while sitting on two stacked wooden platforms.

While the morning breeze was still cool, Surat, Teju, and I went up to the hall, lined up in a row in front of him, and synchronized our movements to his. Despite being close to seventy, far older than the rest of us, he moved with ease. He was still supple and commanded our attention, and I recognized the yogi I had met and loved. I relished the time alone with him, away from Angela and our hectic life in Paris.

Certain of good news on my return, I was disappointed to find my job still hadn't come through, but did my best to stay focused on work despite the uncertainty. With each passing week, my anxiety heightened. What would I do if the new company didn't hire me after all?

On our next call, Trevor said to Fiona, "So have we lost Joelle?"

She was quick to respond. "Oh no, no, no. We're waiting for the paperwork from legal."

He offered to make the right contact and push for my case.

As the dark days of January turned into the grey light of February, I stopped waiting for an answer. To allay my tension, I sought out Chinese massage: an intense form of therapy that left me black and blue in the shoulders and thighs from "trapped energy." I showed my bruises to Angela, and she suggested I reduce the frequency, but I ignored her. I believed in the healing power of medicine from China, Babaji's home country, and needed to tame my thoughts.

In mid-February, six weeks after my return from India, the head of the Nortel HR department in France called me into her office and announced my transfer. I could hardly believe it. She had received my new contract honoring the eleven years I had already worked. All she needed was the signature of the Sales President. My heart sank. We had once had a serious disagreement, and since then, our interactions had been muted. Now he held the keys to my future. She was close to him, so I asked her how she thought he would respond. Her face opened into a smile. "Of course he'll sign your paperwork."

She was present when he authorized my transfer and

wished me well. I thanked them both effusively. They might have been surprised by my behavior, but they didn't know how much I needed this second chance. I had almost lost everything and was determined to set my priorities straight. Starting with expressing gratitude and embracing life's many different blessings—not just the ones in the yoga school.

27

BOUND

On my first day at the new company, I made a deliberate effort to greet each person I met with a smile and an extended hand. "I'm Joelle from Nortel." I had never been so friendly but didn't take anything for granted. The new opportunity had been hard-earned, and I needed to seize it fully.

The office was bright, my commute down from ninety minutes to forty-five. The new job infused me with profound enthusiasm. I would no longer hide behind Arun's charisma and spiritual powers.

My new colleagues smiled back, and after I repeated my introduction several times, one of them said, "We know."

Of course: all new faces at that time came from Nortel.

Fiona led the combined department, and Trevor, who was based in the UK, reported to her and was my new boss. He called regularly to check in on me. At first I struggled to tune into his South African accent and asked him to repeat every other sentence. I worried he would be offended but had no choice; I needed to make coherent responses. He maintained his upbeat jovial approach and seemed relaxed even when it took two weeks for me to get a computer.

The job I had at Nortel was filled, so he asked me to focus on merging sales data from the two companies' different systems. I welcomed the challenge and worked with the conviction that I would be retained. With the prevalence of mismatches and errors, there was plenty for me to do, and I found my purpose.

Angela, who had watched my recent travails with her characteristic reticence, said to me, "You're lucky with work. You'll always have a good job."

Her words were positive, and I appreciated her confidence, but felt she was drawing an implicit comparison with her own struggles to secure a competitive physiotherapy internship.

I worked from the office more often than before, and Arun behaved as if nothing had changed. He went to City Yoga in the morning, returned for lunch, then spent the afternoon watching television before lying down and traveling to the other side for a couple of hours. He had always had a sweet tooth, but since the accident he had lost all restraint. If he wasn't drinking beer with lunch, he had a can of Coke, followed by a pint of vanilla ice cream. Leaning into the couch, legs crossed over the glass coffee table, he struck the ceramic bowl in a repetitive rhythm. If that wasn't enough, he got up for a candy bar.

I couldn't watch his eating habits without saying anything. "You're going to become diabetic!"

He looked at me like I was a nuisance and kept eating.

By summer, Trevor asked me to come to Guildford, the company's European headquarters southwest of London. Eager to make a good impression, I wore a new taupe suit, my hair held up in a bun. I waited in a corner of the vast reception hall, my laptop bag at my side. From the far-left automatic doors, a tall man with greying hair and glasses glided across the hall, repressing a smile. He looked kind, and I was instantly relieved. He was nothing like I had pictured him. Based on a colleague's comment that he was not only tall but broad, I had imagined a blond-haired man with a bulging belly and ruddy complexion. But Trevor looked gentle and scholarly. I could work with him. He welcomed me, took my hand, and leaned in for a quick kiss.

At the end of a long day I looked out from the round attic window of my hotel room in a Victorian mansion. Manicured gardens and forests spread before me. I hadn't expected to be in such a beautiful natural setting and relished my time alone; the luxury of the plush bed with starched sheets, the warm shower and floral-scented body wash. A feeling of peace and independence took hold of me.

Trevor introduced me to a complex spreadsheet with unknown functions and asked if I could replicate it for this year's sales plan.

"Yes." I had no idea how I would do it but wasn't going to trouble my new boss with teaching me Excel.

At the end of our meeting, he leaned back and said, "It's so good to finally have someone to discuss these things with. It's been ten years since I've been able to speak to anyone about sales compensation."

His expression of genuine appreciation surprised me. How fortunate that the expertise I took for granted captured his interest.

I would be leaving the next day, and he offered to take me for dinner. I was nervous about having enough topics to talk about, but as soon as we sat at our table in the pub, he commented on my CV. "How did you learn all those languages?"

There were only three—English, French, and Spanish—and I explained that French was my native tongue, and I learned Spanish at school. He seemed fascinated. I had never met a senior corporate leader who was so down-to-earth, and was pleased to start on a positive note.

We made it through dinner with sufficient conversation, and back in Paris I said to Arun, "I think I'll keep my job."

"I told you. They won't find someone like you."

All those years, he had advised me to stay put when I wanted to leave; maybe he had been right after all.

Later that summer, Trevor informed me that the company had decided to hire analysts in India, and I would be their manager. I had made considerable progress with integrating the two data systems, but it would take time and effort to sort through ongoing issues. The new team, along with a few analysts in Europe, would support the processing and correction work. Working independently had felt like a vacation after a decade in management, but my current job wasn't permanent, and I was glad for the new role. At my first assessment in September, Trevor rated me as "successful" and added that next year, with my team, I would reach a higher level. I couldn't see that far ahead, but his optimism was encouraging.

After interviewing twenty-five candidates, I hired five and planned to meet them at the Hyderabad office, in Central India. Before traveling, I returned to the UK to work with another colleague and didn't spend much time with Trevor, but when it came time to say goodbye and he shook my hand, I was struck by the sadness in his eyes. Perhaps someone he loved had died.

My trip to Hyderabad showed me a different side of India— modern buildings with air-conditioned offices and luxury hotels —distant from the green hills, swamis, and daily chanting of Rishikesh. By the end of the week, I thought I had made a good connection with the team of analysts and they understood their new responsibilities well, but as soon as I was back in Paris, I received an avalanche of phone calls every day. Different team members asked about the same point, as if there was no communication between them. Despite multiple repeated explanations, the pattern continued for weeks. I struggled to stay on top of the mountain of work. Then the unplanned absences started.

I focused on what I had to do and didn't give Trevor much thought until he called one day and spoke in a low tone. "I haven't heard from you since you got back from India. You've gone so quiet. I don't know how to help."

I was used to working for remote executive managers who wanted the job done with as little hassle as possible and hadn't even considered alerting Trevor to the situation. I was surprised by his reproach and decided that if he wanted to hear about problems, I would bring up so many he would soon ask me to stop and understand my initial reserve.

From then on I shared all unresolved issues, however minor. Far from showing the impatience I had expected, he listened and offered advice with his usual cheerful demeanor. Trevor made me realize that I could reach out to someone and didn't need to bear all my burdens alone. By the middle of spring I had regained enough mental clarity to adopt a time management system. I could no longer meet the demands of both my corporate job and City Yoga just by working harder.

With my new focus, I also realized I was carrying too much. The City Yoga lease was up for renewal for another three-year term in December, and I had to make a decision six months earlier. If I didn't send a formal letter to terminate the agreement in June, the lease would renew automatically. We had been in business for over eight years, and never quite broke even. For the first time in my career, I cared about my job. Trevor and I collaborated over the phone, and I spent long hours at work to achieve the best results. I was proud of the broken process I had turned around with my international team.

Angela was also developing in her profession. She had started a physiotherapy internship and reduced her hours at reception. While our arrangement had remained informal, I had to shoulder an increased burden, and decided to speak with her.

The next time I saw her at the school, I stopped her on her way to the massage room. She sighed and dropped her bag by the reception desk.

"Can you sit down for a minute?"

"I need to get ready."

"It won't take long."

She glared and took a seat.

"My new job is taking a lot more time. I can't get through all the work here by myself. I need some help."

She pursed her lips. "What do you want from me?"

"Can you help with some of the accounting when you're here early. I can show you how to do it."

"I don't have time. I'm already doing everything I can here. Sorry if it's not enough, but I can't do more."

I hadn't expected such an unmitigated refusal, and didn't know what else to say.

She swung her bag over her shoulder and continued on her way.

My mind reeled at her callousness. I paid her rent and expected more understanding, or willingness at least to discuss the situation. She knew better than anyone how Arun's deteriorated state compromised his abilities. She was only here for herself, and I wished she had never walked into the school. I rested my forehead in my hands and massaged my temples. Maybe it was time to rethink the business. Owning a yoga school had been my dream since university when I discovered TM, but since my near job loss, my priorities had shifted. Nine years was a good run, and even though we hadn't made a profit or recovered our initial investment, we had developed a regular clientele and kept the business afloat. In December our rent would increase again, making it even harder to make ends meet.

If I had only myself to think about, I would end the lease. But what would happen to Arun without the school? How would he spend his day? City Yoga was the reason he left home in the morning. Without a business to open, he would stare into endless hours of emptiness. I dreaded a return of his days of alcohol-induced torpor punctuated by outbursts of rage. Even if he no longer had the energy and presence to manage the school, I feared what would happen to him without it.

One Sunday afternoon, after we went for a walk in the Bois de Boulogne, I opened the discussion before he could turn on the television.

"I'm so busy with my new job. I asked Angela to help but she refused."

He crossed his ankle over his leg and held it. "I can help."

"I know you want to, but it's hard."

Long sunbeams shone through the door-windows onto the wooden floor. He stared straight ahead.

I took a deep breath. "Arun, I'm thinking about stopping the school. Sending a letter in June to end the lease."

He turned to me immediately. "Why would you do such a thing?"

"We've had a good run. All these years. But we still don't make money. Angela's moving into her new career..."

His lips parted, and his eyes looked stricken. "I don't want to let it go."

I drew in closer. "But do you really enjoy it? Many times in the afternoon, you don't even want to go back. I have to ask you to."

"I enjoy it.'

He repeated my words, but I couldn't tell if he meant them. "It was my dream too, but I just don't know if I can continue like this."

His eyes glistened, and tears ran down his cheeks. I had only seen him cry once, in Fontainebleau, after meeting his spirit parents for the first time. He choked on his words. "Don't do it, Jo. Please don't do it."

The following Saturday, after we'd had lunch, and Arun had retired to the living room, I spoke with Angela about the possibility of closing the school.

Her eyes opened wide. "But what will happen to me?"

"You'll find work somewhere else."

Alarm seized her face. "It's not that easy."

"Look, what do you want me to do? The school isn't making money."

"But it was your dream."

"Dreams change.'

She shook her head. "It's so sad."

I hated it when she descended into melancholic anguish and offered no practical solutions.

She narrowed her eyes. "I think Arun is turning people away. He's so quiet. He doesn't even look up when people come in. It's just rude."

I sighed. "What do you want him to do? Stay at home?"

She thought for a moment. 'What about asking Vanessa to work with us?'

Vanessa was our newest instructor. In her early twenties, she was exceptionally poised and calm. Angela had interviewed her and insisted we hire her.

"That will just add more cost."

Her tone rose as she met my eyes. "We have to try something. You're not seriously thinking of closing, are you?"

"I spoke with Arun about it, and he started crying. What would he do if we closed?"

"But you would tell me, right, if you were going to do it? You know my whole income comes from there."

Her spew of emotion—her very presence in our life—

though it balanced Arun's void, felt like a noose around my neck. If I tried to move, it would choke me.

A few days later, we woke up to the news that Osama bin Laden had been found and killed—close to ten years since 9/11. Arun, who still followed world events closely, told me he had worked on his capture on the other side. I didn't doubt his travels took him to the heart of the fight between good and evil, but how he had intervened, how he operated in a parallel space, I didn't understand.

While I was still pondering whether to give up the City Yoga lease, Silvia, our former client whom Arun had once identified as Angela's sister, called out of the blue while I was on a bus. She had stopped attending classes since meeting her partner and giving birth to her daughter, and I hadn't heard from her in a few years.

Her upbeat voice hadn't changed. "I know it's been a long time. I've been so busy with my daughter. But she's growing up now, and I'm thinking of opening a yoga center. I love yoga so much. You remember how regular I used to be? I miss it."

I looked out the window as we crossed the Pont de l'Alma. "Of course. You're part of our history."

"I was wondering if we could chat. Maybe you could give me some tips."

Before I could respond, her voice broke up, and she said she'd call back another time.

She exuded cheerful energy, and I was eager to hear what she had in mind. Perhaps her call had come at just the right time.

But as the days passed with no sign from her, my inspiration to effect change dissolved. The window to cancel the lease passed, and my personal guarantee on the rent renewed for another three years. The intricate bonds between Arun, Angela, and me remained untouched. I lacked the courage to take the difficult step I knew I must.

28

SOUL MATE

In the autumn, I prepared for the inevitable rent increase and sought out additional sources of income: outside instructors who wanted to rent our hall, and a package of heavily discounted classes marketed through Groupon. Over three hundred deals were bought on the site in twenty-four hours, and though it was a one-time hit, we netted a few thousand euros. We hovered on the edge of profit, and every intake helped.

One afternoon while I was working from home, Angela called me in a panic.

"You have to come see this."

I was in the middle of a task and tried to tame the impatience in my voice. "What is it?"

"He's been trying to change the printer cartridge for forty-five minutes. There's ink everywhere. It's a complete mess."

I couldn't ignore the situation and told her I would be there as soon as possible.

"Hurry, please."

I sighed and pulled myself away from what I was doing. Why did she turn everything into a drama?

I was at the school ten minutes later and found Arun facing the printer, his hands dyed in bright ink. He was completely focused and didn't look up.

"Thank God, you're here." Angela pleaded with her eyes.

"Stop, you're going to break it," she said, then turned to me. "He's been trying again and again, but look what he's done."

The desk was covered in blotches of colors. I almost felt sorry for her. "Let me handle it."

She stepped away, and I went over to him. "Love, what's happening?"

"I can't get the new cartridges to fit."

"Let me take a look."

He left me his warm seat. I extracted the blocked cartridges and reinserted them so they clicked into place. "There you go."

He looked at the printer in a daze. "Thanks."

I fetched a wet washcloth and wiped the ink from his hands, then the table.

"I just couldn't get it."

"I know. It's confusing. Don't try so hard, love. Let me help you."

As students filtered in for the evening class, Angela said, "Just in time. Can you imagine if they had seen us like this?"

I welcomed them with a composed smile, then went to find her in the massage room. The scent of geranium and rosemary filled the cloistered space.

She stared at me. "Do you really think he should be working here?"

I held her gaze. 'Where else do you want him to go?'

"Let Vanessa be with him at least."

"And how do you think we'll pay for that?"

She shrugged and turned away. It was easy for her to dream up ideas; she didn't have to settle the bills at the end of the month.

"Even if we could afford it, this is his place. There would be no yoga school without him."

Later when Arun and I walked home together in the darkness, I clasped my fingers around his and felt a surge of love for him. He had suffered so much. "You'll tell me if you're tired, right, love?"

He dropped my hand. "I'm not tired."

AROUND THAT TIME, he started talking about having a pet. He first mentioned a bird, but I said I didn't want a caged animal. Then I caught him browsing pictures of puppies on the internet and asked him what he was doing. He said he wanted a dog.

"We're not getting a dog."

He kept quiet, but a few days later, he said, "I want the smallest dog ever."

"You mean a Chihuahua?"

I couldn't help looking over his shoulder at images of puppies, but hoped his interest wouldn't turn into a plan. Just in case, I brought up the difficulty of keeping a dog in an apartment and the demands of pet ownership.

"I want one," he replied.

"Do you really mean it? It's hard to look at puppies and leave them at the store."

"I don't want to leave them."

"But I already told you we can't get a dog. Not here. Not now."

He stared at me without a word, his gaze soft as a child's.

"We'll see, okay? I can't think about it right now."

While he repeated the same demand every few days, I did my own research. If we ever went ahead with his crazy idea, we would get a female. Easier to handle.

I spoke with Mom about his new fixation.

"Why does he want a dog?"

"I don't know, maybe he's lonely."

"A dog is a lot of work."

"I know. But maybe we can manage it."

"If you get a dog, choose a short-brown-haired one. Low maintenance."

He eventually won me over with his single-minded focus, and we went to a pet store on the banks of the Seine near the Louvre. The Chihuahua pups were in a floor-level cage. They bounded all over each other, but now that I saw them up close, I didn't feel drawn to them. I wandered away and spotted two fluffy white balls staring at us through the bars of their raised cages. "Oh Bichons! I know these dogs." I had once spent a day with one when a friend brought hers along for a visit. "So sweet."

Immediately a sales assistant came to open the gate and placed a tiny female in my arms. She clung to my shoulder as I held her. Arun would have preferred the larger male with a curlier coat and gentle eyes, but seeing us torn, the assistant nudged us to the female. We bought her on the spot.

At home she pranced on the rug in the living room and followed us around. I couldn't think of a name and settled on Annie. Angela came to see her and marveled at the tiny creature.

I smiled. "I named her after you."

She scrunched her lips. "I don't want the dog named after me." She placed a finger on her chin and thought for a moment. "She's so white. Why don't you name her Lily?"

MY CORPORATE WORK was even more demanding now that we were in the new financial year. Trevor and I had met briefly in the summer and worked together in a close office. I had picked up a hint of his smell and normally would have shrunk away to create more space between us, but there was something unexpectedly familiar and sweet about him. My attraction was unexpected. Yes, this man had been kind and helpful to me—the first person outside the yoga world I had felt close to—but he was a friend, nothing more.

As he had predicted, my team and I had been recognized for our valuable contributions to the sales teams, and I was determined to keep up our achievements. When one of the analysts had to take unexpected leave, my responsibilities increased, and I traveled to Guildford twice to pick up the work.

On my second visit, at the end of a long day of work, Trevor suggested a quick meal at the American diner near the office. We sat at a booth with red vinyl seats while sixties rock music blared over the loudspeakers. He thanked me for my repeated visits.

"It's no problem."

"It must be hard on your family."

"My husband is a businessman."

His gaze drifted to the diamond solitaire Arun had bought at auction. "Oh yeah? What kind of business?"

"He invests in India."

"Does he travel a lot?"

"Only a couple of times a year."

"That's not too bad then."

The conversation veered to him, and he mentioned a potential job abroad. I couldn't imagine losing him at this critical point in my career and felt relieved when he said he had refused.

After our burgers arrived—his meat and mine vegetarian— I felt I should tell him something about myself. "My husband is my soul mate."

I had expected his eyes to light up, but instead, his lips parted slightly. "Is that right?"

Maybe I had hit a sore point.

On a Saturday after my return, Arun, Angela, and I were eating lunch together when he opened a tiny bottle of chili tincture. The stopper was unfastened, and half the contents poured onto his shrimp dish, dying the rice the color of rust.

"You can't eat that," I said.

His current physical complaint was intestinal pain. I had taken him to a specialist who had asked him questions, then berated me for speaking over his silence. She ordered a battery of tests, but there was nothing visibly wrong, and he continued to ignore my suggestions to modify his diet. He craved intense flavors and bought the spiciest chili sauce he could find on the internet. He ignored my warning and scooped up some rice.

I pleaded with him to stop, but he kept on eating. I couldn't watch him harm himself deliberately and went to take his plate away, but he held on and tugged it back.

Angela glared at me.

I sat down in defeat. "You're going to get hurt."

"Leave me alone."

He finished his food with his usual uninterrupted mechanical movements, but no sooner had he left the table than he doubled over in pain.

"I told you." It was exasperating and sad to watch his obstinate destructive behavior.

He left Angela and me to clear the dishes, and when we were done, we returned to the empty dining room.

"He's not well, is he?"

I shook my head.

"What are you going to do?"

"There's nothing I can do, is there?"

A shaft of diagonal light pierced the gap between the white curtains. She looked toward the window. "If something happens to him, you won't want to be with me."

My throat constricted at the suggestion of his death. Imagining a life without him brought on immediate overwhelming anguish. His presence was my anchor, my link to the other side, life beyond death. His warm embrace and penetrating gaze was confirmation that I was loved. I didn't know whether I would survive without him and preferred not to think about it.

I took a deep breath, quelled the onset of tears, and turned to Angela. "I never said that."

She held the moment, her shining grey eyes resting on mine.

I insisted, "We'll be together after ..." I couldn't say it.

She picked up her bag, walked to the entrance hall, then stopped and glanced through the glass-paneled doors to the living room. Arun was lying quietly on the couch.

"What is he up to? Sleeping again?"

"He's not sleeping. He's traveling." So many years with us and she still didn't understand his spiritual work.

I closed the door behind her.

Arun had said to me long ago, before we opened the school, that I would be in my sixties when he died, too old to look for a new partner. He seemed happy with his assessment, but I had dismissed it. I didn't look forward to living out my sixties alone. Surely a yogi who had mastered physical longevity would live beyond his nineties. Now at seventy-one, he was already unwell, and though I had tried to reassure Angela about my commitment to her, I didn't see a future together. In all my visions, there was always a time when she would be gone.

29

FRIENDSHIP

In October Trevor and I met at the annual sales conference in Berlin. For the first two days, I saw little of him, and on the final evening I wore my only dress for the celebratory party. The color of eggplant, it was fitted at the top, then flowed down to my knees. It was gift from Mom, and I was wearing it for the first time. Trevor walked over to where I was standing with a couple of colleagues and commented on how lovely we all looked. He glanced down at my shoes, and I wondered if he had expected me to change out of my daytime flats, but they were my only formal shoes.

I didn't see him at the party—dancing and karaoke didn't seem to be his thing—and after a couple of hours socializing with our sales colleagues, I left, not expecting to find him standing outside in a group of suited men. He smiled and introduced me, and I joined them for a few minutes before excusing myself. He did the same, and when we reached the dimly lit entrance hall, he asked if I'd like to have a cup of coffee. I declined—it was past eleven.

The final morning the executives rallied the troops in a

large auditorium. Trevor took the seat next to mine, and as we listened in silence, I breathed in his scent over the whir of the air conditioning. This time I wasn't surprised.

The conference was over, and we ate lunch together before boarding the bus for the airport. We fell into an easy chat about what we wanted to do before our flights, and I imagined us in deep conversation. When the driver announced our destination, Trevor shot up. He had followed me onto the wrong bus, unaware that Berlin has two airports. He rushed out without a word, and I was jolted out of my daydream.

At the airport I wandered in and out of shops in a daze until I finally sat down with a cup of coffee and poured out my feelings in my journal. Around the time of the team discussion with our client about the future of City Yoga, I had prayed for a male guide. It was unusual for me. Dad was a mystery to me, and I tended to contact him only out of need; Arun was all I had ever wanted in a man. But he had changed, and I needed help. I sensed it wouldn't come from Mom, who hated him, or Angela, who looked up to him. Trevor was my friend, but why did I feel so distraught when we separated?

I reached home late that night. Arun was asleep, and I undressed in the dark and slipped into bed. As my back touched the sheet I felt a warm dampness, and an acrid scent rose to my nostrils. I bolted up, lit the bedside lamp, and threw open the bedding. A dark-rimmed yellow stain marked the sheet. "Yuck. Lily peed on my side of the bed." She was curled up at his feet. He opened his eyes, and I spoke as if he were fully awake. "Help me change the sheets."

He worked in slow silent movements until we were done. I changed my clothes, returned to bed, and turned away from him. He wrapped his arm around me and went to sleep holding me. How had he ignored the smell?

. . .

ANGELA CALLED one afternoon just after Arun had gone to open the school. "I sent him back."

"What happened?"

"His breath smelled of alcohol."

"He probably had a beer at lunch and forgot to brush his teeth. I'll remind him."

She lowered her voice. "Some of the students commented."

"So what do you want me to do? I'll speak with him tonight."

"Maybe he should stop coming here in the afternoons."

"I told you already we can't afford to pay someone to do reception work. We can barely keep up with the teachers' salaries and rent."

"You sound annoyed. I was only offering a suggestion."

On Saturday, he was browsing images of dogs on the computer again, and I asked him what he was doing. He said he was looking for a mate for Lily.

I stood by his side, hands on my hips. "We are not getting a second dog. Besides, how can we breed dogs in an apartment?" As it was, he had taken no initiative to walk Lily until I insisted we each do so once a day.

I stepped back and watched his steady focus on the screen, his thick fingers over the mouse; his white hair pulled into a short ponytail, thin and sparse; white stubble on his jaw. On Mom's last visit she had suggested he get a haircut, so he would look younger.

"Why do you care anyway?"

"I care about you."

I was used to his long hair, the beard that framed his face. I wrapped my arms around him, and as he held my wrists in his warm hands, I kissed the top of his head.

It was late in the afternoon, and Tao would soon be here. As if on cue, he let go of my arms, and his head dropped to his chest. When he lifted it, his face broke into a gentle smile. He went to the bedroom, and I took his seat and buried my face in my hands. Arun's departure still put my belly in knots.

Tao returned in a fresh set of clothes. "What is it, Jo?"

"I'm sad, that's all."

"Do you want me to stop coming? I can leave and never come back if that's what you want."

"That's not what I'm saying."

"Then?"

I sniffled.

"He'll be back in the morning. You know that."

The front door clicked behind him, and I swallowed the lump in my throat. I missed the man who woke up ready to chat and comforted me with his insights. The brain injury had consumed him. I closed my eyes and prayed. *God, help us find each other again. Heal us from this nightmare, and bring Arun back to life.*

I WALKED to my seat at the Thai restaurant slightly self-conscious in my shape-hugging sweater dress, wondering what Trevor thought of my new style. After the sales conference in Berlin, almost two years since I'd joined the company, I had visited my family in New York and asked Saby to take me shopping. For the first time since I moved to Europe with Arun fourteen years earlier, I spent money on myself and selected fashionable outfits. Saby insisted on buying me heels.

Trevor didn't say anything, but when we selected the same dishes and picked up food from common plates, our friendship entered a new level of closeness.

I would soon be leaving for Hyderabad to work with the team there, and when we were back in his car he asked me once again about my decision to travel over Christmas; one of our colleagues had expressed concern. I couldn't reveal my reasons—how traveling and spending time alone in a hotel relieved the pressure valve of my life at home—but we ended up speaking about religion.

He said, "What religion am I? You don't know."

"Jewish?"

"I'm Christian."

Oh yes. Why had I said Jewish? We were in Guildford, not New York City.

Although I had already been to Hyderabad twice, he asked me to send him a message when I arrived. Texting him from my hotel room felt special; someone on the other side of the world cared about me.

On my return in January, we met in Guildford for a couple of days. I wrote figures on a whiteboard while he sat behind me.

"You can't see," he said.

I turned back to him. "I can see."

He spun in his seat and faced the window outside. "What about that tree over there? Can you see that?"

"I can see the tree."

"But what about the branches? Can you see the detail in the leaves?" He took off his glasses. "Try these."

I felt awkward putting on something of his, but took them and gazed outside. The green leaves appeared in vivid detail and varying shades. "Yeah, that's better."

"Get your eyes checked. You need glasses."

I had had a laser operation to correct my severe myopia five years earlier, and while I managed without glasses, over time low levels of myopia had crept back in. I had resisted getting glasses, but Trevor was right: I couldn't see as well as I should.

In February we were invited to a leadership conference for senior leaders: three days to motivate us to drive better results for the company. I looked forward to the time away from regular work. On the first evening we ate with a colleague, but on the second we stayed at the conference venue to catch up on work. We made brief attempts to read emails after a full day of talks and exercises, then admitted that we were exhausted and left to find a restaurant in Maidenhead, the town where I had lived for a couple of years before moving back to Paris.

In the dark winter evening, I could hardly recognize the High Street where Arun and I had spent almost every weekend. At twenty-seven, I had felt so lost, confused about our struggles, yet hopeful that we would overcome them. Twelve years later, I was older, more in control of my life and self-assured.

We searched for an appealing restaurant, but didn't find any and settled on a pub where we found a table in a quiet corner away from the bar. The space was cast in a warm glow. One man sat in a corner with his laptop, while a couple spoke quietly with their fingers interlaced across the table. I waited for Trevor while he went to buy drinks, and when he returned, I told him I would pay for the food, to keep things balanced.

He grinned. "What do you mean 'balanced'?" He motioned between us. "What's going on between us?"

I feigned surprise. "Nothing is going on between us."

That evening, we spoke about our families for the first time, and I realized how little we knew each other and how much more I wanted to know about him. He had become the person I was most interested in.

He noticed I was cold and offered me his suit jacket.

"I'm fine." I smiled. "What would people say if they saw me wearing your jacket?"

He shrugged. There were windows to the street, and colleagues could walk in. I didn't want to take a chance, but was surprised that he didn't care.

After the conference, I could no longer deny that given the opportunity, Trevor and I would be more than friends. But I was married, and the forbidden, adult love I felt for him had to remain shut in its box.

Back at work, I applied the motivating messages from the conference and took an interest in colleagues outside my immediate department. I was inspired to see beyond my own job and asked them what they did and what problems they faced. I engaged in conversations over lunch, where I made a point of sitting with others rather than eating alone. I developed a regular group of office friends, with a solid core of women who stuck together.

That winter, whether I wanted it or not, love gave me a surge of new life. Arun was still there, but he wasn't everything to me anymore.

I decided to buy something I had wanted for a long time but thought I couldn't afford: an iPad. Arun and I went to the Apple Store on a Saturday after closing, and I asked for the newest model. He said he wanted one, too.

"No. You can't have one. This is just for me." I was irritated with his sudden demand when this was something I had waited years to buy. "We can't afford two."

He looked at me with surprised hurt, but I didn't care. He had been in command for sixteen years; this was my time.

Then he asked to go to the pet shop.

High on the victory of my new purchase, I didn't want to say no again. Better to get this obsession out of his system.

To my relief, there were no Bichons on display that day. I stepped out to take a call, and when I returned, he was staring at a glass cage at the back. A fluffy white ball was pressing its snout against the pane with a defiant expression. Arun demanded the puppy, which didn't even look like a Bichon, and when I hesitated, he said, "I know him. We had this dog in Tibet."

A sales assistant released the puppy from the cage, and

Arun carried the small male to the counter at the front. "I never thought I would find him again."

I tried to argue that we couldn't afford another large expense —not so soon after the iPad—but he ignored me. He was smitten and didn't take his eyes off the tiny ball of fur. Whatever Arun saw in him, this dog couldn't be the reincarnation of a former pet; but I wondered if this creature would lift him out of his misery.

As if driven by a power outside myself, I handed over my credit card for payment.

We introduced the puppy to Lily in the entrance hall of the building, and once she had accepted him, we let them loose in the living room. They quickly took up positions on the rug, howled, and engaged in a circular chase. I had never seen this boisterous play and tried to restore order, but Lily was fixated on her new companion and ignored me.

The enormity of what I had done hit me, and I sank into the sofa. The glow of the halogen lamps in the dark night cloistered our space. How had I ignored my better judgment and succumbed to his madness? How could we possibly manage two dogs?

Arun watched with amused interest, oblivious to the gravity of the situation. My belly knotted. "We've made a terrible mistake."

"They're just playing."

I didn't see it that way. Our delicate peace—my newfound sense of control—had vanished in a flash. Panic rose like acid inside me, and my body felt heavy and limp. Sobs broke through. "This is crazy. I should have never listened to you. Our life will never be the same again."

Arun finally took notice of me. "Why are you crying like this? What do you want from me?"

I couldn't answer.

"A divorce? Is that what you want?"

The sharp edge in his voice shook me. He hadn't said the D-word since the fight in Paris before we moved to Valbonne.

My voice rose through the tears. "I never said I wanted a divorce."

"Then?"

"It's just so much."

The next day, I told Mom what we had done.

Her tone was sharp and high. "You did what?"

"I just told you we got another dog."

She sounded dismayed. "Why?"

"Arun wanted it." I couldn't tell her about his breeding plans.

"I don't understand. You were going to get one short-haired brown dog. Now you have two high maintenance, white dogs."

"I know. Things changed."

She sighed. "I don't know what to tell you."

Angela came to see him, sat on the couch, and ran her fingers through his fur. "He's adorable. In an ugly way."

I smiled.

"I'm only joking." Then she looked at me. "Why did you name him Benny?"

The name had come to me as soon as we left the pet store. "I like the sound of it, I guess."

She looked concerned. "It means 'son,' you know."

"I know."

"So you think this dog is your son?"

"Hey, maybe he is." What did she know.

As spring came, my world had expanded, and I was floating. One late afternoon, standing in the shadows of my bedroom, I passed the pink and gold framed mirror hanging on the wall. It had been in the bathroom of my parents' apartment and reminded me of my childhood. A voice sounded in my mind. *If you pursue this man, it will be complete dissolution. Everything you have will be destroyed. No part of your life will remain untouched.* In an instant I saw the carefully constructed edifice of my life come crashing down. Arun, Angela, City Yoga, the elders—they would all go. An unknown, unseen world would emerge from the rubble. It was a tantalizing prospect, but was I prepared to demolish everything?

30

THE MASK

We couldn't afford to pay another person to do reception work, but Vanessa increased her presence and arrived early before her evening classes of her own accord. I called the school one afternoon while she was there, and Arun answered in a gruff voice. He sounded distressed, and I asked him what the matter was.

"These women just walked right past the desk. They didn't even stop to check in. I had to shout at them."

"I'm sure they were just busy talking."

"Here's Vanessa. She wants to speak with you."

"I heard him telling you about my students."

"Yeah, he sounds upset."

"He called them 'bitches.'"

"He said that?"

"Yes, as they left the desk. I think they might have heard him."

"I'm so sorry."

"It's all right. But I told him to keep his voice down."

She was gracious about it, but he was out of control. His

intestinal pains wore him down, and his mood remained low. Even his interest in sex, a former constant, had receded.

One evening in May, I was doing the bookkeeping at the school and found some cash missing. There had either been a mistake in recording payments, which was unlikely, or someone had lifted a few bills. Neither Angela nor Vanessa would ever take money from the drawer, so it had to be someone else. But who? No one else worked at the desk.

When Angela emerged from the back, I shared my quandary with her.

She shrugged. "You should check what Arun's doing. He keeps his eyes glued to that computer. I don't know what he's up to, but he's not helping the school." She delivered her judgment. Then walked away.

Always Arun.

I was annoyed at her tone and implication, but she had given me a lead, and on Saturday, I sat at the desk with him. He was staring at the computer, one hand on the mouse, the other pressed into the table. The screen was filled with bright objects.

"What are you up to?"

"Nothing."

I didn't recognize the website he was browsing. "Arun, tell me what you're doing."

"Nothing."

I touched his arm. "Come on, show me."

He shook me off. "Leave me alone."

"I can't. You're at the office. Now show me what's going on."

He emitted a loud sigh, glared at me, and rolled his chair back.

I drew in closer. "What is this?"

"You bid for stuff."

"What stuff?"

"Cameras, phones."

"How are you paying for this stuff?"

He didn't say anything.

I froze. "You aren't?"

He looked at me as if I were an overbearing parent.

My jaw dropped. "How could you?"

He looked away.

I tried to tame the crescendo in my voice. "When you know we're struggling to pay the bills."

I forced myself to breathe and held back a surge of tears. His illness, insidious and intractable, was taking over.

I touched his arm again. "You've got to stop."

"Okay, I will." He closed the browser window, then pushed the keyboard and mouse away. "I can't seem to do anything right around here."

He got up and walked over to the bowl of candies he had put out for clients. He picked up a toffee, unwrapped it, and popped it in his mouth. Then he sat on the bench, chewing and gazing straight ahead.

I took a deep breath and turned toward him. "We're working here. We can't use company money for ourselves."

He left shortly after our exchange, and I stayed to welcome students for the second class. Our bank statement arrived in the morning's mail, and I ripped it open. There were eight different payments to Groupon and a bidding site; two thousand euros of charges. His underhanded activity was even more advanced than I expected. I was beside myself.

When I arrived home, he was cooking lunch, and I thrust the statement in front of him. "What's this? Did you know what you were doing?"

He picked up the pages and squinted at the entries.

"This is stealing from our own company."

I left him and went to the living room, sat on the couch and buried my face in my hands. What on earth was he thinking?

A few minutes later he came to see me, and I pulled myself up. "Arun, this is very bad." My voice quivered. "You are forbidden to use those sites and charge items on the school account. Promise me you'll never do it again." I stared into his eyes.

"Okay, okay." He stayed rooted in place and looked at me.

Pigeons cooed on the balcony, and warm spring light penetrated the room.

"The food's ready."

I shook my head. "I don't want to eat."

He went to fill a bowl for himself and returned to eat in the living room. His metal spoon striking the ceramic bowl accentuated the emptiness. He seemed removed from what he had done. Blood flowed to my head, and hot tears poured down my face.

As he finished eating, the intercom rang, and he went to answer. "It's Angela." As if she needed an announcement. He stood in front of me and stared. I ignored him and gave in to my distress.

"Will you stop?"

"Why should I stop?"

"Please don't let her see you cry."

Why shouldn't she see me cry? He wouldn't get his way this time: not now that I had his attention.

When Angela arrived, she took one look at my bloated eyes and rushed to my side. "Why? What happened?"

I spoke between panting breaths. "It's Arun."

She touched my arm and waited for me to explain. A fresh wave of pain squeezed my chest. "Sorry you have to see me like this. Arun asked me to stop, but I can't . . . I, I can't stop. I feel so sad. So, so sad."

Arun watched us wordlessly.

She pulled a tissue from her bag and gave it to me.

I wiped my nose and took a breath. "Don't you want to eat something?"

"No. Let's go out."

My head was sore, and I felt exhausted. "Now?"

She looked determined. "Let's go shopping. You said you need new sandals."

The last thing on my mind was footwear, but I didn't want to stay in the apartment with Arun either. Where was the wise teacher who had taught me the art of physical longevity? What was the point of long life if it was to buy cameras and gadgets he didn't need?

Angela led us to the bus stand in the glowing afternoon. She didn't ask questions—perhaps she felt like she didn't need to after warning me about him—but I wished she did. Perhaps if we unpacked the elements that didn't make sense, we could piece together clues about our strange life with him. But she focused on the necessities of living.

The bus was filled with Saturday shoppers, moms with kids, teens bursting with life. My eyes swelled, but I swallowed the tears and tried to merge with the flow. My mind kept returning to the missing cash. Had he taken a bill here and there? I couldn't know for sure, but there was no other explanation.

Angela guided me to a small shop she knew well. It was filled with shoe displays. My heart wasn't in it, but I didn't want to be difficult, so I picked up a pair of platform sandals. She scrunched her face. "You're not used to heels."

She found a dainty pair of low-heeled black-suede sandals with a bow across the toes. Too cute and not my style, but she suggested I try them, and I went along. I was ready to end the expedition and left with them in a bag.

On the bus ride back the weight of our aloneness pressed in on me. Angela had tried her best, but shopping hadn't worn the edge off my pain. She squeezed my hand when we parted in front of her building, and I trudged up the street toward mine, the same trajectory she had taken that first time with Tao. I had survived the searing pain of that night, but nine years later the aftershock was still there. There was no safe place in our triangle.

When I reached home Tao had arrived and greeted me with a smile. I recognized him from the show of emotion that was now rare for Arun. He asked about Angela, and I told him she was at her place. He wanted to see the contents of the box, and I held up a sandal.

"They'll suit you." He smiled, then clasped his hands and stared at the empty television screen.

"What are you up to?"

"I'll go soon."

"Already?"

"You want me to stay?"

"No, I just thought . . ."

I wondered how much he knew. It felt awkward complaining to him about Arun.

"What is it, Jo?"

"Nothing. I didn't realize the time."

Being alone with Tao cheered me up a little, but after he left the sinking feeling returned to my belly. I hadn't eaten anything since breakfast and found some leftover shrimps and rice from lunch. It had been a while since Arun's absence on a Saturday evening brought on such a rush of anxiety. My mind wandered to a conversation I had with Mom last time I was in New York. She had taken me for coffee at a new penthouse restaurant with a stunning view over the Hudson River. We sat on comfortable low chairs in the dimly lit room, and she asked about Arun.

"He's not doing well. He's abrupt, uncommunicative. And he suffers from the most terrible stomach pains." It was difficult to reveal his true state, but I could no longer hide that there was a problem.

Her expression was calm. "Does he still drink every day?"

"Yes. That's never changed." I paused. "I don't think it ever will."

"It's not good for him. After his accident."

"I know. But he won't listen. I can't reach him anymore."

"I'm sorry, sweetie." Her cup made a gentle clink as she returned it to its saucer.

I stretched my lips into a thin smile. "What can we do? He used to be so talkative and friendly. Everyone at the school gathered around him. It's not like that anymore."

"Who you see now is the real Arun. His social mask fell after the brain injury."

After what he had done, I couldn't stop thinking: had Arun become dishonest? Maybe she was right, and underneath the veneer the real Arun was anti-social, wasteful, immoral. I watched three episodes of *Friends* before going to sleep.

The next morning, I was drinking coffee in the dining room when he returned. The white curtain thinly veiled the window. He glanced at me and took his usual place at the table. Although the table was round, his seat felt like the head. I went to get him a cup of coffee, then we sat in silence. His face was smooth and clean-shaven. His soft brown eyes more alive. I wanted to believe in him but couldn't make sense of his actions. I willed him to speak about the prior day, but when he stayed silent, tears streamed down my face.

He turned to me. "What is it?"

"I'm just so sad."

"All this crying, Jo, for two thousand euros?"

"Yes, Arun. All this crying for two thousand euros."

By Monday morning my mind had cleared, and I turned my attention to the practical matter of recuperating the funds. I asked our family doctor to send me a note about Arun's brain injury and his consequent inability to make sound buying decisions online. She was reluctant at first, but when I relayed his uncontrolled buying spree, she relented. I closed his online bidding account and called our Groupon sales representative to ask her to cancel all his open bids and terminate his account. She said she didn't have the authority to do so, but when I mentioned the doctor's note, she agreed to help—only because she knew me. By the end of the day I had recovered about half of the inappropriate charges. The rest would be deducted from the company's start-up debt to us.

I was traveling to Guildford the following week and needed to take care of one more matter before I left. It had been years since I had visited Angela at her home. Our relationship was shaped by Tao's appearances and her changing moods, and I left her alone in her space, but I had something to say to her, and we agreed on a visit late Sunday morning.

I squeezed a path through the shoes lining her entrance hallway and the clothes piled on the wall hooks. The main room was overflowing: stacks of papers on the desk; towers of books on the floor; mounds of shoe boxes. A cacophony of objects vied for every inch of space. Angela lay on the futon propped up on pillows. The curtains were drawn, leaving only a chink of light. She looked exhausted.

I stood at the foot of the bed. "Are you okay?"

Her voice was drained. "I'm fine."

"Can I open the curtains a bit?"

"Sure, go ahead. I was reading, and the light was blinding me."

I parted them a foot and returned to the small couch which faced into the room away from the bed. "Can I sit here?"

"Anywhere you want."

The energy in the room felt oppressive. We hadn't spoken since our shopping trip, and I didn't know what was troubling her. Did she still enjoy Tao's visits? If I didn't have something to tell her, I would have left. She stared into the distance, the late morning rays illuminating her eyes. I sat at the edge of the couch and turned to face her. "You seem upset."

"I can't believe what Arun did."

I met her gaze. "Yes, I wanted to speak with you. I'm sorry I made such a big deal about it. I was in shock." I offered a weak smile. "I feel better now."

"I don't."

"I don't think he realized what he was doing."

She folded her arms across her chest. "He's a grown man. He should know better."

"He had an accident." I was repeating myself again.

I took a breath and continued. "I spent most of last weekend crying, but it's out of my system now." Her sullen expression didn't budge. "I've forgiven him." There, I'd said it.

Her eyes rested on mine. "Well, I haven't."

Maybe she would have said more if I had encouraged her. But it was too late: our time to draw closer had passed. I wasn't ready for her to take a stance against him; I needed her to stay in place just a while longer. Tomorrow, I would be in the UK.

31

APPLE BLOSSOMS

Trevor leaned back in his seat at the pub and scrutinized my face. "I don't know if I'm supposed to notice these things, but did you get a new piercing?"

I adjusted my black cardigan over my new pink dress, crossed my arms on the table, and smiled. "Yes, you can." I had the piercings done with Saby on a shopping trip downtown and had been worried about Mom's reaction, but she hadn't noticed. No one had, apart from Trevor.

He gave my ears an appraising stare. "It looks good."

He had already noticed my dress that morning when I stood behind him in the cafeteria line. It was such a radically different look from my sober suits that he had said, "It's nice to see you like this." I had decided against too many changes at once and left the heeled pumps from Saby in my suitcase.

The following day we met with Fiona, his boss, who had come over from Ireland to work with us. She invited us to join her for dinner that evening, but Trevor declined. I was traveling for work and couldn't refuse, but was disheartened to have run out of opportunities to socialize with him. Before he left the office, I spontaneously invited him for breakfast at my hotel the next morning, the last time we could meet before my flight home.

He thought about it for a moment. "Yes, that would be nice."

With my bags packed fifteen minutes ahead of our meeting time, I decided to take a walk around the gardens in bloom, but when I reached the main entrance of the hotel, he pulled into the drive, and I followed him into the parking lot.

He stepped out of the car and said, "You're early, too." Light flooded his eyes, and enthusiasm animated his lips. He took my hand and planted a kiss at the edge of my mouth. I was happy to see him, but he glowed with joy.

We took a table for two in the dining room, and after we had served ourselves from the buffet, it occurred to me that I hadn't informed the hotel about my guest. I mentioned my oversight to Trevor, and he grinned. "They would never ask a lady about her breakfast companion."

I had toast, jam, and an egg, but he seemed famished, and ate a full plate of English breakfast, then got up for another. I was glad the meal was such a hit.

When we were done, he said, "You've done so well in this job, you must be pleased."

"It's been good."

"What's next for you?"

"I don't know."

"Did you have a chance to speak with Fiona yesterday?"

"Not really. We didn't talk about work."

"You should. She knows how talented you are."

He removed his glasses and placed them on the table next to my sunglasses. Kindness radiated from his eyes.

"I want to show you something," I said.

"What is it?"

"Come with me. You'll see."

As I left the table, he handed me my sunglasses. "You forgot these."

We stepped out onto the veranda facing the gardens. The smell of cut grass and roses filled the air. He shielded his eyes from the sun and looked out. "This is stunning."

"Wait until you see the trees."

I led him to the grove of apple trees near the entrance. We stepped into the tapestry of pink blossoms, and he started to comment, but the sudden dimness and chill of the shade caught me by surprise, and I moved to the entrance. As I crossed into the light, I extended my arm. He took it and held me.

"I'm sorry," I said.

"Don't be sorry."

We stood just outside the apple trees, his arms wrapped around me, my head in his chest and hands in the crook of his back. I worried for a moment that someone would see us hugging in the sharp sunlight. Then I abandoned the thought. It was a huge risk to cross the confines of my world with Arun and the elders; strangers didn't matter.

I looked up and kissed the scar at the base of his neck. "How did this happen?"

He flinched. "It's a long story."

We were so close, yet I knew so little about him.

He drove me to the office, and when my taxi arrived to take me the airport, his face looked pained as he waved good-bye. Already it was difficult to part.

BEFORE I BECAME involved with Trevor, transgression had seemed impossible: I would remain faithful to Arun for life. Now that I had stepped outside the bounds of my marriage—

with someone who didn't even know yoga—I was fallible. I had left the world of the saved.

Yet if the elders could see us from the other side, then they knew about Trevor. And if they had let him come so close to me, he must have their blessing.

For the first time, Tao's appearance on Saturday left me indifferent. I craved the freedom to be myself and welcomed Arun's departure for an evening. He could have his love; I had mine. The knot in my belly was still there, but I was finding my way around it. I had opened a parallel door in my life, and it was thrilling.

By Sunday morning, it occurred to me that Trevor and I didn't have a plan to see each other again. He was about to leave for a two-week holiday, and our communication would be limited. I felt adrift and asked Arun for a puff of his marijuana. I had tried it only once, when we first moved in together in Fontainebleau, with no noticeable effect. I didn't know how to smoke, so Arun took a long drag, held it in his mouth, then exhaled into mine. The hot fumes burned my throat, and I let them out through my nostrils. At first, I felt no different, then a focused lightness enveloped me—nothing so exceptional that I would spend so much to burn my throat, but that day I wanted to blunt the sharpness of separation.

Dad invited me to attend an art gallery opening with him. It was rare for us to spend time one-on-one, especially in such a beautiful, relaxed setting. The windows of the mansion were cracked open, letting in a gentle spring breeze, and we wandered through the high-ceilinged, parquet-floored rooms, commenting on the exhibits. My resentment for him dissolved. He might not be the dad I had wanted—one who upheld moral principles and showed me the way, one who was interested in me and whose constancy I could rely on—but he was the dad I had. I let go of my childhood expectations of him; he was flawed, but so was I. Perhaps for the first time I found myself loving a genuine man, not one I had conjured up in my imagination—and being loved in return. I didn't need Dad to be the man of my dreams. He was demonstrative, holding my shoulder, kissing me. I accepted him and began to forgive him.

On his return from holiday, Trevor created an encryption system so we could exchange email messages privately at work. Whenever the jumble of letters arrived, I couldn't wait for the next free moment to decrypt his messages. He wrote about his feelings in a way that was passionate yet real. He didn't recognize me from a prior life, but chose me in this one.

We had long conversations after work, speaking while I was on the train, then on my twenty-minute walk home. I hadn't spent so much time on the phone since my teenage years. If we still weren't done by the time I got home, I would stand outside the building, indulging the heady sensation of speaking with someone who had my complete attention and desire.

Dad's business partner, who lived in our studio down the same street, caught me on one of these sidewalk conversations. I smiled and nodded as he passed. He might have suspected me and told Dad, but what if he did? The discovery would surprise them all.

Each time Trevor and I spoke we added threads to the weave of our relationship. He was outside the spiritual world I had inhabited for the past seventeen years—not the man I would have ever expected to fall for, but a genuine friend and companion. My mind was lit to the potential of a new life though I didn't have a clear picture of what it would be.

I made a point of attending Vanessa's Friday evening relaxation class along with our clients. I tuned into her voice and followed her instructions.

"Let's start on all fours. Take a deep breath and arch your back. Exhale and round your back." Her calm steady voice, her presence and teaching, lifted me from my personal concerns. This was what our clients experienced; the reason they came to us. To unburden themselves in the space of an hour. It felt good to be a student, for once.

Despite the tension and uncertainty of that time—the future vague and unknown—it was the spring of all possibilities. The blossoming of all the seasons I had missed since marrying Arun.

32

THE WHEEL TURNS

The renewal of the City Yoga lease came to haunt me. Had I known a year earlier how close I was to entering another world, I would have ended it when I still had a chance. Now only six months into the new three-year term, the higher rent ballooned our running costs, and Arun's lack of engagement made it harder than ever to attract new clients. As I had done in the early years, I supplemented the monthly revenue with my savings. If only I had followed through on my reasoning, I would have been released from the cycle of debt. I couldn't sustain it all anymore; something had to give.

I called Arun and Angela into a meeting on a Saturday after the clients had left. She had reluctantly agreed to stay behind, and they sat at opposite ends of the teak bench. I leaned in and looked at them like a teacher delivering a lesson. "The school didn't make enough money to pay the rent this month."

Right away, Angela scowled and looked away.

Arun got up for a sweet, popped it in his mouth, and returned to the bench.

"I had to use my savings again. We can't continue like this."

I paused. "Last year I asked you if we should give up the lease. You both said 'no.' Now I'm paying the price."

She turned to look at me.

He blinked with cultivated gentleness and remained silent.

"Angela, you're not covering the reception hours you used to before your studies. I can't afford to pay your entire rent on top of supporting the school."

She hadn't been expecting this turn in the discussion and sat up, her eyes wide.

"You used to do twenty hours. Not anymore."

"What am I supposed to do? Where will I live?" She acted like I was kicking her out.

My voice rose more than I intended. "You can do what everyone else does and pay some of it."

"Where do you want me to get the money? With my salary, I don't have anything left at the end of the month."

I had anticipated her reaction and didn't rush in to fill the space. The computer fan whirred, and Arun stared at his lap in silence.

Angela turned to him. "She wants me to pay."

He looked at me. "Don't ask her, Jo. You know she can't pay."

It felt like we were parents discussing our child. I straightened my shoulders. "Well, neither can we. We've invested all our savings in this place. If we fall short again, we won't be able to save the school. Then what will happen?"

She pouted and stared at the floor.

For too long I had bent to their wishes, but I didn't need to anymore. I felt Trevor's invisible presence behind me and spoke the words I had held back for years. "I'm asking you to contribute, that's all. It's only fair."

She spoke without looking up. "I don't have the money."

"Then maybe it's time we give up this place."

She looked at me as if I had suggested burning it. "You don't mean that."

"Why not? What do you want me to do? Do you think money grows on trees?" My temples started to pound. How could she be so selfish?

Her pitch rose as she addressed Arun. "She wants to close the school. What will happen to me? Where will I go?"

"Let's see, let's see."

I shuffled paperwork on the desk. Angela got up, slung her bag on her shoulder, and said she had to leave.

Arun didn't speak on the walk home, but after we sat down to eat, he looked at me with his deer eyes. "Don't close the school, Jo."

I held my voice steady. "What do you want me to do?"

"Angela has her massage work. Don't ask her for more."

"She gets paid for that. We don't owe her rent on top."

"I'll help. Tell me what to do."

"Love, you don't even focus on the reception work when you're there. You play games on the computer. It's not helping."

When Angela and I next crossed paths at the school, she looked somber and hardly uttered a word.

In July, when I went to Hyderabad for work, I left them in charge with Vanessa's help. I returned two weeks later and was standing in the kitchen when I had an uncanny experience. I sensed Trevor's presence, turned, and saw him standing in the door jamb—as real as if he had been in the room. The vision only lasted a second, but the feeling that he was there persisted.

It was a Sunday morning, and I would have preferred to relax at home after the long trip, but I needed to go to City Yoga to check on the accounts before the work week started. Arun came along, and though he was aloof, I appreciated the company.

I sat at the desk, rifled through the post, and separated two white envelopes from the property agent. The first letter contained the rent check I had mailed before leaving; the second demanded immediate payment before the end of the month. I logged into our online bank account and gasped.

Arun looked up from the marketing brochure he was perusing. "What is it?"

"The July rent check bounced, and we only have forty-five hundred euros in the account." Not nearly enough to cover the current month's rent plus the upcoming payment for August. I planted my elbows on the desk and buried my face in my palms. "What are we going to do?"

"We'll make money again in September."

"But we can't start the new season two rents behind." Rivulets of panic wended through the pit of my belly. "This shouldn't be happening. Something has to change."

I transferred ten thousand euros from my savings account to the business account and drafted a proposal to sell the business.

MOM CAME to visit in August and witnessed Arun sitting on the couch, day after day, watching terrible television programs. When she saw him with a tumbler of amber liquid in his hand, she raised an eyebrow and motioned for me to follow her to the balcony. The summer sun warmed our skin, and she looked at me with concern. "He shouldn't be drinking." She hardly ever voiced her disapproval since his illness.

"I know."

She was right, but I had stopped trying to control his drinking. I had other concerns. After she left, I would be going to the UK to meet Trevor.

While Mom was with us, Gabriel got in touch with Arun, seven years since he'd walked out of the school. News of his renown in the yoga world had filtered to us from our clients. He had achieved guru status, drawing hundreds of students to his outdoor classes. We were happy to hear from him after so long, and Arun invited him and his girlfriend over for lunch. We prepared roast chicken and vegetables and greeted them with smiles and embraces. Gabriel had filled out a bit, but still had the same carefree expression. His girlfriend was a movie actress with a cherubic face, and he was proud to introduce her to us. I was delighted to see him again.

As soon as the couple settled on the couch, Benny and Lily jumped up to join them, and she stroked their fur. Gabriel's knee touched hers, and he rested his hand on her leg. Arun offered them wine, then returned to the kitchen to complete the meal preparations. Mom had met Gabriel after we opened the school and joined in the conversation. His girlfriend was smitten by the dogs. "They just radiate love."

When it was time to eat, Mom left, and we joined Arun in the dining room. I saw immediately that he had been drinking. Our guests declined his offer of more wine, and he filled his balloon glass to the rim. We sat at the table, and as he raised the glass to his lips, he spilled wine on his shirt.

I was sitting to his right and stared in his direction. "Be careful."

He looked ahead with a blank expression. "I'm sorry."

We ate in silence for a few minutes, then Gabriel's girlfriend commented, "This food is delicious."

Gabriel smiled and added, "Yes, very good."

We hardly spoke for the rest of the meal, and Arun's eyelids drooped. I nudged his leg under the table and startled him awake. He emitted a loud belch and apologized again. Gabriel and his girlfriend looked down into their plates, and I tried in vain to catch his gaze. When he finally glanced in my direction, he seemed unaware of my discomfort and radiated content-ment—as if all he had wanted was to see Arun and introduce him to his beautiful girlfriend.

After the meal, I offered our guests coffee in the living room, and Arun excused himself to go rest in the bedroom. I hoped Gabriel might take the opportunity to ask me about Arun's state, but he made no mention of it, so I asked about his teaching. He told me about the huge crowd that had come to his outdoor class in the Champ de Mars gardens around the Eiffel Tower. "All those people raising their arms just because I told them to." His eyes shone. "It was incredible."

I found his fascination with his mass following disturbing and tried to redirect his attention to Arun's compromised state. "We don't get big crowds at the school."

He ignored the suggestion and went on to tell me about the retreats he led in Sri Lanka. "Have you ever been there?"

I shook my head.

"It's amazing. Wild. Untouched." He clutched his girlfriend's knee and looked into her blue eyes. "We're planning to get married there next year."

I asked him if he had read *Yoga Body,* a recently published book about the international origins of modern yoga practice. In an exhaustive academic study, the author, Mark Singleton, explained how yoga postures, which are mostly absent from older Hindu texts, originated in India at the turn of the twentieth century from a combination of local and foreign influences. Gabriel had wondered about this question himself and asked to see the book.

When we ran out of topics, I finally told him Arun had been unwell.

He nodded with an impassive smile. "It was good to see him."

I couldn't tell if he didn't understand the situation or if he didn't care, but after he left, I felt a deep sense of loss about Arun.

I went to check on him in the bedroom. He seemed to have just woken up and tottered around the bed. His thin hair was raised from his scalp, his gaze unconfused, yet he seemed wired. It must be Tao.

"You look tired. Why don't you rest some more?"

He ignored me and hobbled toward the bedroom door. "I'm going."

"You can't go like this."

"I have to see Angela."

"You don't have to do anything. You can barely stand."

The smell of stale alcohol laced the air.

"You can't walk."

"I'm fine."

"You're not fit to go anywhere. What's the urgency?"

As he moved past me to leave the room, he banged his head on the edge of the open door.

"See! I told you."

He put his fingers on the wound and examined the streak of blood for a moment, then continued to the bathroom.

I called after him. "How will you walk there?"

It was pointless trying to reason with him, and I went to wait in the living room.

When he emerged from the bathroom, he walked straight to the front door and held the knob. "I have to go."

Ten minutes later Angela called me. "I sent him to take a shower. What happened?"

I told her about Gabriel's visit, Arun's drinking, and his physical state when he woke up. "He insisted on seeing you."

I was glad he was with her. At least I wouldn't have to worry about him for a night.

A FEW WEEKS LATER, when autumn had set in, Angela came over and asked to speak with me alone. It was an unusual request as she mostly kept to herself. Arun was occupied in the living room, and I guided her to the bedroom on the opposite side of the apartment. She sat on the bed near the window, and I settled on the other side, near the door. Night had fallen, and the overhead light cast an amber glow. She pressed her hands into the comforter and looked up after a moment. "I don't know if I can do it anymore. It's become so difficult to be with him."

She didn't need to elaborate: Arun was distant, heavy in his pain, not in the mood for sex (thankfully for me) yet disturbed by his own lack of desire. As irresponsible as ever. But I wasn't expecting her to speak about Tao and trained my ears for hidden notes.

Her pitch rose. "I can't take it. He's changed so much. He hardly speaks when he comes over." Her distress sounded like a child's—how she seemed to me before she became my husband's lover.

My tone was cool. "Or is it you who's changed?"

"Don't say that. I do everything I can. But nothing seems to matter." She looked into my eyes and blinked. "I want to take a break from him."

Her words shook me. Of all the elements that might move, I had least expected it to be her. She had been forging her own path for years, but her link to Tao—and to Arun and me—ran deep.

She had voiced a more skeptical view of Arun's intentions only once, that past summer. He must have done something to elicit her displeasure, and when he had gone, she had turned to me and said, "He's lucky to have two such young women with him."

I was shocked by her implication that we were victims somehow. "What do you mean? We were both adults when we met him. And we chose to be with him."

She shrugged and kept silent, but her insinuation bothered me. Did she think we were like those two teenagers in California? Manipulated by an older man? She was wrong: we were free and old enough to determine our fates.

Now she came to tell me she wanted out. But if she left him, Arun wouldn't cope. He depended on her, whatever she meant to him. And I had major financial obligations at City Yoga until we closed the business. We needed planning to dismantle the links.

"What will we do at the school? What happens when Arun sees you there every day?"

She pinched her lips. "I need my work, you know that."

"I know, but what about him, how will he feel?"

What did she expect from me? She had benefited from our arrangement for years, a regular income, her rent paid. She couldn't just decide to leave Tao one day and keep everything else intact. As much as I didn't want to admit it, Tao and Arun were one unit, two halves of the same circle. And though I resented her presence and her dark moods, she'd been the closest person in my life; I couldn't cope with him on my own.

33

THE OTHER SIDE OF MY SOUL

When I spoke with Trevor—when I heard his voice on the train or while walking home—I felt alive. I held onto his words, the timbre of his voice, and told him what I had kept secret for so long: my yogi husband channels a spirit who visits a woman. Trevor rewarded my trust with understanding and expressed concern about Arun's involvement with spirits.

But when I told him Arun insisted on holding me or being held every night, he stopped at my words. "You still sleep in the same bed?"

"Well, yeah. We haven't separated."

"I didn't start a relationship with you for you to continue to sleep with your husband."

His message—simple and sharp—hit to the core. Arun and I no longer had sex, but why was I still sharing a bed with him?

That night, I laid the futon mattress we had for guests on the living room couch. When Arun asked what I was doing, I told him I needed my own space. He didn't insist and retired to the bedroom.

In that one step, I untied the knot that held us together. There was no going back now.

For the first few nights, he accepted the situation, then one evening, he stood outside the bathroom while I was brushing my teeth. He waited for me to finish and said, "When are you coming back to our bedroom?"

"I'm not."

As I brushed past him, he smiled and touched the side of my buttocks.

"Stop." His gesture, though gentle, was sickening, as if what I missed was sexual contact with him.

I walked across the hallway into the living room. He stood still by the double doors. The space was perfectly quiet; only the halogen ceiling lights broke the darkness.

I turned to him and spoke in a steady voice, "I'm leaving you."

"You don't want me anymore?"

"I want to be on my own."

"You want a break?"

I fixed my eyes on him and kept my voice soft and firm. "I want to separate."

He paused for a second. "What should I do? Should I go back to India?"

"If you want to."

"I'll go to India. Book my ticket."

"I will."

Satisfied with the solution, he turned away and went to the bedroom.

In the silence, I dialed Angela's number, later than I would have normally phoned. When she answered, I said, "I'm leaving him."

She held the weight of my words. "What happened?"

"Nothing. It's over."

I had done what I needed to do—for myself and for her. Leaving him was an obvious consequence of his behavior, yet a victory at the same time. She of all people would understand.

ARUN DIDN'T PROTEST my decision. Once I left the bedroom and escaped his clutching embrace, whatever had held us together for years broke. I focused on practical matters, booked his flight in two weeks, and didn't consider the death of our eternal, otherworldly love.

Angela came over one evening and handed me a small bag and an envelope. "These belong to you."

I opened the envelope and found my diamond heart pendant taped in the center of the card with the words: "Here is your heart. Never forget. Love, Angela." The bag contained the rest of the jewelry I had given her when we first met.

"Thank you."

"When is he leaving?"

I told her mid-November, and she stood there for a moment in silence. Just a few weeks ago, she had wanted to leave Tao. Arun's departure should be a relief, but her mood was heavy, and she didn't stay long.

Now that I no longer cared, Tao stopped visiting.

I had let go of Arun as a man and as a lover, but I wondered about the couple we had been. Why had a spiritual seeker in her early twenties been paired so long with an older yogi holding the keys to immortality? If we were soul mates, why had our relationship broken?

In a quiet moment before he returned to open the school in the afternoon, I declared, "You're not the other half of my soul."

He looked at me with tender eyes, "Then who is?"

Another time, I knelt beside him and placed my hand on his heart. "I want to ask you something."

He turned and listened.

"Was I really your wife in a past life?"

He pressed his hands on mine. "Yes, Jo, you were. We were very close."

"Then why are things not working out this time? The school didn't succeed. Angela's not happy with Tao. It's been difficult for so many years."

He held my hand for a moment, then let go. He had no answers to my questions, but the next day he said Babaji wanted to speak with me on Sunday.

The Babaji? After all these years?

I believed in Arun's channeling but was stunned that the most enlightened master of all time would visit me. Thoughts fluttered in my head in the days leading up to the meeting. It seemed odd that Babaji, who had been absent and unreachable, would make an appearance now; but who was I to question his ways? If he was the all-knowing, perfected spiritual master, he would see right through my heart.

Trevor told me to be careful.

"I'll be fine," I said, unable to contain my excitement.

I didn't know what Babaji liked, so I bought macarons and loose-leaf tea.

Late Sunday afternoon, when Arun said it was time, he sat cross-legged on the couch, diagonally to my left. The darkened room hummed with the faint background noise of the radiator and appliances. I felt my heart beating and focused on the rhythmical flow of my breath.

Arun closed his eyes and dropped his chin to his chest. When he lifted it a moment later, a veil of light emanated from his face. He spoke in a rough guttural tone as if it was a struggle to form sounds. "Mother Joelle."

I bowed my head, then pushed the plate of macarons toward him. "These are for you."

He took one, gobbled it in a single bite, then ate another with the same ravenous gesture. His display of primal hunger surprised me, but before I could offer anything else he said, "Something to drink."

"Tea or coffee?"

"Alcohol."

"Beer?"

"Something stronger."

I was unprepared for his request. Tao and Udo drank copious amounts of alcohol, ideally spirits, but I didn't expect Babaji to do the same. "Let me see what we have. I'll be right back."

I dug out a small bottle of rum from the kitchen cupboard, poured the amber liquid into a tumbler, and brought it to the living room. I resumed my cross-legged seat. A gentle pulsation transfixed the space.

The being inside Arun drained the glass in one swig, then addressed me. "Will you stay with him?"

I fixed my gaze straight ahead. "I cannot."

"Why not?"

"I . . . I can't."

"He loves you."

The air felt heavy and still. I remained immobile, concentrated on slow breathing, and waited. Before long, Arun's head lolled to one side, and the visit was over.

The light was gone from his face, and he blinked and looked at me, "What did he say?"

"He asked if I would stay with you."

"And what did you answer?"

"I said I can't."

I rose and left the room.

Whoever had passed through Arun had focused almost entirely on pastries and alcohol. He was nothing like the grand master of my imagination: a man beyond sin and the travails of the world. A master yogi was supposed to be omniscient or, at the very least, read minds, but this one knew nothing of my private longings. If I hadn't felt a palpable change of energy, I would have thought it was a trick; Arun making a final dramatic case for himself. But if not Babaji, then who did Arun channel?

I recounted the experience to Trevor, and he said, "Why did you buy him sweets?"

"I thought he was an honorable guest."

He didn't think Arun's practices were benign.

"I've known about Babaji for years from books. Before Arun even mentioned him. Some say he even taught Jesus in the lost years."

"I'm just glad you're safe. Be careful."

Whoever had come to speak with me, it had been a dismal disappointment.

ANGELA CAME to say goodbye to Arun a couple of days before his flight. I stayed in the dining room but could overhear their voices across the hallway. They exchanged a few words, then he asked her for something.

"How much do you need?" she said.

"Anything you have would help."

"I can give you two thousand. That's all I have."

"That will do. Thank you."

He was preying on her, as he had on me; but how could he do it to her, when she had so little to give? How could he take all her savings?

They moved to the entrance, and as she was about to leave, she dropped her voice, but I could make out her words. "I want to ask you something. Did we really know each other in a past life?"

His eyes would have been tender, warm. "Of course. We

were good friends. Same as now." He would have held her in his arms and reassured her, once again, that she was loved, cherished, always had been.

I felt sorry for her and didn't want to hear any more. I left the dining room and went to sit on my bed.

On his last day at City Yoga, Arun said goodbye to whatever long-standing students happened to be there. We hadn't announced his departure, but our clients understood that something had shifted. We left after the midday class and stepped into the November chill, as we had so many times before. On our walk home—the last we would ever take together—I felt a sense of purpose, like a mother bringing her child back from school.

He finished packing that evening. His green duffel bag bulged with all the items he had amassed in the last two weeks: every phone we had ever owned, digital cameras, floral-scented body shampoos—all the things he wanted to have in India. He even took my 35mm camera from high school, but I didn't argue. I didn't need the camera; I needed him gone. Surprisingly, he showed no interest in the large brass statue of Ganesh that we kept at the top of the bedroom bookshelf; his chosen deity looking down from his seat with care and protection was left behind without a word. When he was done, he circled his bag, searching for something.

"What is it?"

"I can't find my platinum chain. It was just here."

He had just gone to retrieve it from its safekeeping place—how could he have misplaced it already? We retraced all the steps he had taken, but it didn't appear.

"It must have been taken to the other side," he said after a few minutes of searching.

My brow creased. "How is that possible?"

He hunched his shoulders.

In theory, anything was possible, but why would an entity

from the other side reach into the material world and take a heavy necklace? It made no sense. Still, how had his most expensive possession—fashioned just for him, and paid for with my hard-earned savings—disappeared now, on his last day in Paris? I felt drained.

He zipped his main bag, then packed his backpack. As he was about to place his mobile phone into it, I held out my hand. He had bought an iPhone behind my back, knowing I would oppose the unnecessary expense. He stopped in his tracks and met my stare.

"You won't need that where you're going. It will cost a fortune if you make calls with it there."

He paused for a second, then flung it across the table. I caught it on the other end. He wouldn't need his links to France in Rishikesh. It was a small but important victory.

We left the apartment early the next morning and waited on the sidewalk for his taxi to arrive. In all his trips to India over the years, I had never accompanied him to the airport or gone to pick him up on his return, but this was his last journey. As the taxi circled the Etoile, the Arc de Triomphe aglow in the sun's rays, we sat in silence and gazed out of our respective windows into the morning sky.

I stood in line with him at his departure gate until I could go no further. As if unaware of our parting, he focused straight ahead. I touched his arm. "Take care, okay?"

He realized what was happening, reached his arm around me, and brought his lips toward mine. I turned away, and he grazed my cheek. Still holding me, he said, "Wait for me. Promise me you'll wait."

I shook my head and whispered, "I can't."

He let go and merged with the crowd.

I didn't need to rush home and found the metro back into the city. Waiting on the platform I inhaled the crisp morning air. On the train, the chug of the wheels rocked me as I looked out the window. Low-level buildings passed by like a film. The perfect orange disk of fire rose in the distance. The world was impervious to the end of my marriage. As it should be.

I had nothing more to say to Arun: I had told him everything I ever wanted to say.

34

THE D-WORD

Night had fallen pitch black, but when I entered the school, I felt a warm enveloping welcome. Vanessa looked at me with knowing eyes, and asked how I was doing.

I attempted to smile. "I'm fine."

The evening instructor didn't know Arun had left, but she picked up on the mood immediately. She led me to the back room and held my hands. Her green eyes bore into mine. "You haven't . . . separated?"

I nodded.

She held my gaze and assured me we would get through this time.

Rachel had been one of my earliest students, and we had a good rapport. I felt a particular closeness with her, and back in the summer she was the only one I had told about my desire to sell. She arrived that evening and sat on the bench, waiting for class, and said, "I'm always up early. You can call me any time."

On my first evening alone after Arun left, the women surrounding me filled the space.

Then Angela walked in from the cold. The grey fur of her coat collar hugged her neck. She glanced at all of us, walked over to the bowl of candies, and turned to us with a stricken expression. "Who's going to fill this now?"

No one uttered a word. Vanessa met my eyes for a brief moment, and Angela marched to the back. She had never liked the display of sweets, insisted it didn't fit the image of a yoga school. Now it was the first thing she noticed.

Vanessa took over many of the gaps Arun left at reception and generously offered to work a month without pay. Only Monday evenings remained unattended, and I asked Angela if she could cover the hour before I left work, but she refused, citing a regular appointment she couldn't move. I turned to Rachel, who lived close by. She agreed to open on Monday afternoons and register clients for the first class. I offered her payment, but she declined. She wasn't helping for money, but out of care and friendship.

A few days after Arun left, I called Angela one evening. I wasn't looking forward to the conversation, but it was important. Trevor saw it as a critical step to breaking Arun's stronghold. When she picked up the phone, her voice was as tight as a bolted iron door.

"I can't keep paying your rent," I said. "I'll pay for all your hours of reception. Same rate as the others, but you need to cover your own rent."

The door creaked open. "I don't think I can do that."

'Well, neither can I.'

"I need time to work things out."

"How much time?"

"Three months."

"I'll cover November and December, but you need to start paying from January."

"Then I'll move out."

"That's up to you."

I offered her a discounted rent, and she reluctantly agreed. When our conversation ended, my mind swirled in the mixed currents of relief and indignation. After all I had done to help her over the years, she treated me like a malicious stranger. If she hadn't been forced upon me as Tao's wife, we would have never been so close.

As SOON AS Arun reached Rishikesh, he called me as if I had never mentioned separation. "When can I come home?"

"You can't." I felt like saying, "This isn't your home," but didn't want to provoke him.

He had wanted to buy a massive 3D television in Paris for months, but I kept refusing. It was a huge expense, and we didn't need a more vivid view. It was the first thing he acquired for himself in India, probably at an exorbitant cost, but he was free to make his own decisions now. How he spent his money was no longer my concern.

Every couple of days he renewed his pleas to return to Paris. When his name appeared on my phone, my stomach tightened. I could hear the drone of his voice and feel the pressure of his emotional overtures.

"I miss you. When can I come home?"

"I already told you. You can't."

"I want to come home."

"You are home."

"Why are you punishing me like this?"

"I want to be alone. That's all."

He cried and sniffled. "Why? What have I done?"

I kept quiet, and he settled down.

"I need money."

I was prepared. "Send me the keys to the apartment."

"Then you'll send money?"

"Once I have the keys, I'll arrange something."

Alone in the apartment, I cooked for myself—something I had never done while he was there—and shielded myself from the specter of his presence. At least I had Lily and Benny for company now; especially Benny, who would bark at any ghost.

I went to retrieve the bag of jewelry Angela had given me. I had tucked it away in the hidden recess of the bedroom bookcase, but the space was empty. How odd. I didn't recall moving the bag.

In a flash I realized what happened and called Arun.

"You took the jewelry Angela gave me."

He cleared his throat. "I thought you didn't want them."

"I didn't give it to you."

"I told you when I was packing."

My mind was reeling. "You did not tell me. You stole it from me."

The line was silent.

"How much did you sell it for?"

"I don't know yet."

"Don't tell me that. How much did you get?"

"A hundred thousand rupees."

Two thousand euros. He had stolen my jewelry—everything he could find in the apartment—for two thousand euros. Heirlooms from Mom and pieces he had bought over the years were in a bank safe he didn't know how to access.

After he had been gone a couple of weeks, Trevor asked, "Have you started the divorce process?"

I stumbled in my reply. "We're separated. But yeah, I guess I will."

"What else did you think would happen?"

I had never imagined the word "divorce" applying to me. My parents had divorced after a prolonged separation, but I had clung to the notion of marriage as a lifelong union. Not from the Catholicism of my youth, but from my own romantic and spiritual ideals. My soul mate—the being who already knew me and would complete me—would never need to be replaced. We would live out our days together, doing good. The idea of changing husbands felt like a failure and a sacrilege. I had only just accepted my transgression with Trevor; I hadn't yet thought about how to end my marriage to Arun. But though divorce sounded formal and foreign to me, it was inevitable: the final step I needed to take to secure my freedom.

I asked Dad about a lawyer, and he directed me to Marc Lambert, our all-purpose family lawyer. Then he expressed concern about Arun's intentions. "He can come after everything you have."

I felt confident I would be able to hold my ground. "I hope not. I'll try to settle." Then I dropped my voice. "It's hard, you know."

"I know, Jo. What matters is that you loved, not whether you were loved. Nothing else matters in the end."

I didn't know if I believed his philosophy, but I appreciated his intention.

It took me a bit longer to tell Mom. She had been through so much already during my relationship with Arun, and I didn't want to burden her any more. I finally phoned her from the kitchen one evening and told her I was divorcing.

"I never thought I would live to hear those words," she said.

I held back tears and apologized to her for all the pain I had put her through.

"It's all right, Jo. You don't know how to love in half-measures."

When I told Vanessa, the first person outside my family, I felt like I was practicing the words: "I'm getting divorced."

She looked at me with understanding. "Honestly, I don't

know how you did it all this time." She had been there one morning over the summer when I opened the business email and found that Arun had deleted all the sent messages. Again. After I had told him not to touch that folder. I hadn't been able to stay calm.

The D-word, which had once felt forbidden, almost impossible to utter, grew on me with use. I announced it to my lunchtime companions at work, and one woman's eyes lit up. "Congratulations!"

I returned her gleeful expression and thanked her. She had got it right.

With repetition, the word changed again; it became exciting. Could *I* be a divorcée? It felt risqué and enticing. I would no longer be a woman wed to a man. I would descend from my moral high ground. Enlightenment would no longer be my goal. I was fallible and free.

Before going to visit Mom for Christmas, I emptied Arun's side of the wardrobe and expunged his presence from the bedroom. I selected a few items—his two pairs of leather shoes, formal jacket, a few cotton shirts—packed them in a suitcase and stuffed the rest of his clothes in a huge duffel bag from Saby's university days. The bag would go to charity, along with the large brass statue of Ganesh and a few other Hindu ornaments we had around the house. I didn't want anything to pull me back into his energy.

Next, I decided to have the cotton-candy pink bedroom walls—the sickeningly sweet color he had chosen—painted the palest shade of rose.

The morning after my arrival in New York, I sat at the edge of Mom's bed, with the familiar open view of skyscrapers and Central Park to my right. I leaned in and gave her a hug, and when I pulled back, she examined me for a moment.

"Something's changed. Since you met Arun, a veil covered you. It's lifted now. You feel light."

I held her hand. "Mom, I'm so sorry. For everything I put you through."

She looked into my eyes. "Someday you'll have to tell me what happened."

"I left him. That's all."

She had been through enough. Leaving him was something I needed to do on my own.

Trevor came to visit me for a few days in the new year, and I went to pick him up from the Gare du Nord train station. It was the first time I saw him in jeans, and as we rode on the bus, legs touching, I pointed out famous sights and common places that meant something to me.

On his last day, we were sitting at the dining table, and he asked me if I was a Christian.

"I was born Christian."

"But do you believe that Jesus Christ died on the cross to save us from our sins?"

I had never thought about it like that. When I lived in Paris as a young child, I had gone to catechism once a week, as did most of my classmates. When the teacher told us about Jesus's miracles, I discounted them as stories to make us believe in him. I didn't understand his deeper message, nor the need for an intermediary to his all-powerful father. But in my exclusive allegiance to the father, I had paid a price and lost myself. I needed redemption.

"I want to."

Trevor surveyed the room where I worked, took phones calls, and had eaten so many meals with Arun and Angela. "I sense something here."

I wasn't surprised.

"Do you want me to pray?"

"Yes."

He walked throughout the apartment and prayed in Jesus's name to remove all evil influences from the place.

I didn't know for sure if Arun had left behind bad energy, if he wielded that kind of power; but what he had done, how he had lived, was evil. Channeling Tao, Udo, and Baba—whatever those beings were—he had sought to dominate and control. He had hidden his true identity; for every mask he pretended to remove, another one appeared.

35

UNEXPECTED OFFER

The lawyer Marc advised that the easiest way to obtain a divorce was by mutual agreement.

"What if he was unfaithful for years?"

"We'd still need to prove it, and the procedure would take much longer and cost far more."

He also told me to register our separation at the local police station, mentioning "my husband's abandonment of the marital home."

I went there early one morning. The waiting room was empty, and I was soon taken into an office to record my statement. I explained that Arun had left of his own accord and returned to India, and that while we were married he had threatened more than once to kill me and my lover should he ever find me unfaithful. The words I had found passionate in my youth fell heavily now.

Arun's apartment key arrived by courier, a small item in a thick envelope, and I realized I had omitted to ask him for the fob that unlocked the building doors. He should have sent both without my asking, and though I didn't feel as safe as I would have liked, at least he wouldn't be able to enter the apartment. The key couldn't be replicated without a specific code.

I upheld my side of the agreement and sent him a stipend of three hundred euros a month to cover his expenses in India, then called to ask him for a divorce. I braced myself for his outcry, but after a short pause, he said, "I'll need money."

"How much?"

"I want forty thousand euros, half of the value of the studio we bought together. The apartment is yours from your family."

He didn't claim half our assets, as Dad had feared, only his portion of the joint investment we had made when we first moved to Paris. It was a surprisingly reasonable request, and though I didn't have the money available, I could get a loan for it. I agreed.

"When do I get the money?"

"On the day of the divorce."

"When will that be?"

"I don't know. Could be up to a year. Hopefully sooner."

"I need it now."

"The sooner you sign the paperwork, the quicker it will be."

I had my own request. "I want half of the house in Rishikesh."

"It's rented for two years. I can't sell it."

"After that."

He agreed, but a couple of days later, he called again. His name filled me with dread.

With no preamble, he upped his request to sixty thousand euros and asked for the yellow sapphire ring we had bought at an auction.

I sensed he was pushing me and I needed to hold out. I told him I couldn't do it.

"That's what I need to live the rest of my days."

"What about the money you got for my jewelry?"

"Okay, you can deduct that."

"You can have forty thousand and the sapphire ring."

He agreed.

"And you won't change your mind again?"

"I won't."

"I'll ask Marc to draft the divorce papers."

I breathed a sigh of relief. It was finally happening, and he wasn't resisting it.

"How's Angela?"

My belly gripped. "She's fine."

"She's not answering my calls."

'That's not my problem.'

"Tell her I say hello."

The peppermint green walls of the dining room vibrated. I left my seat and paced. "Don't you know why I left you? Why I can't be with you?"

His voice instantly turned saccharine. "Whatever it is, Jo, forgive me. I will change, I promise. Stop this, and I'll do whatever you want."

"You just asked about Angela."

"I'll never see her again."

My voice rose. "It's too late. Much too late now. It's not just your drinking and senseless spending. It's her." I returned to my seat and stared at the garish walls. "I can never forgive you for bringing her into our life."

"I didn't want to. It was for Tao. You will never have to see her again."

He would say anything to return to his former comforts.

"It doesn't matter now. I can't take you back."

ANGELA LEFT Dad's studio at the end of February, and I gave her keys to him. He had never intended for me to use his apartment for so long, and returning it to him was a reparation of my wrongdoing. The timing was fortuitous as he needed the place and moved there with Lena a month after Angela's departure. At the age of thirty-six, ten years since she walked into our life, she had an apartment of her own in a neighborhood of her choice. The transition she had resisted so much hadn't been impossible after all.

I focused my efforts on selling the school. The personal and financial burden of managing it was too great, and my heart wasn't in it anymore. I spoke to our regular clients about my plan, and one of them sent a promising lead—a businesswoman who already owned a yoga studio in the city and wanted to expand. We chatted over tea on a Friday afternoon, and she promised to get back to me by Monday. On schedule, she called and told me that after serious consideration, she had decided not to pursue the deal. I asked her to make a counteroffer, but she said the price wasn't the problem: to make a profit she needed two halls to hold simultaneous classes at peak times. Her assessment was disheartening.

By March, I hadn't found a buyer, and over our last dinner at his former apartment, Dad made the radical suggestion that I sell the business for free. He argued that it was a huge financial liability and giving it up had a value. I hadn't considered giving up ten years of effort and considerable investment for nothing in return, but he was right. With no taker, I would need to keep paying the enormous rent.

I let it slip to our clients that I was open to any offer, even zero.

Trevor and I met in May for a camping holiday in England's Lake District. I had wanted to go camping for some time but never had the opportunity. I imagined the joy of sleeping in nature, breathing the fresh air, and walking in the mountains. In our week together, the worries and pressures of my life in Paris receded, and the possibility of a different future with Trevor took form. On my return, my decision was clear: no

matter what happened, I would close the business by summer;
I wouldn't reopen for the new season in September.

With no interested party on my side, I contacted the agent
who had signed our lease and managed the property. Negotiations about the rent and arguments over maintenance issues
had strained our relationship over the years, but after I
explained my changed personal circumstances and desire to
close the business, he offered to look for a new tenant. He also
reminded me that if his search was unsuccessful, I was still
liable to pay the rent for the remaining eighteen-month term. I
knew my obligations and lined up a bank loan in case there
were no takers.

In the meantime, the divorce process was underway, and I
had to pay significant notary fees for the documents confirming
the terms of our agreement. I took the jewelry I had kept at the
bank and sold it through the same auctioneer from whom
Arun had bought so many lots.

While I was preoccupied with the future of the business,
Angela strayed further into her own world, and Vanessa, who
often worked at reception after her shift, complained about the
chaos she left behind. Credit card receipts were strewn haphazardly on the desk, and software check-in entries remained
incomplete. "I don't understand why she's doing this."

I shrugged. Her behavior felt careless and spiteful, and I
couldn't make sense of it either. She only ever spoke to me to
express anguish over the sale of City Yoga and press me for
updates.

When I told her I didn't have any news, she insisted. "But
you realize all my income comes from the school?"

"Yes, I know. I'll tell you as soon as I hear something."

One time, after asking her usual questions, which still had
no answers, she lowered her voice. "They say you've met a guy."
She dropped the word like an accusation.

I sighed. "What else do you want to know?"

By the end of May, the property agent hadn't found a new tenant, and I was resigned to paying off the balance of the lease. Then Silvia, our former client, called me out of the blue. I hadn't heard from her since our interrupted conversation two years earlier when she had said she wanted to open a yoga studio. She had the same charming voice, and I could hear her smile. After we exchanged a few pleasantries, she said, "I heard you're selling City Yoga."

"It's time. Arun and I split up."

"I'm sorry to hear that."

"It's okay. These things happen."

"You remember I called you about opening a studio. Things got so busy with my daughter, I didn't get back to you, but I'm still thinking about it."

"Who told you I'm selling?"

"First, Angela. Then a couple of days ago—on my birthday, would you believe it?—Gabriel. He didn't even know it was my birthday. It felt like a sign."

Her exuberance filled the line. Angela and Gabriel—our original partners: I had set them up and considered them family. It felt like a sign for me, too.

Silvia and I met the following Sunday. She walked around the school reminiscing about her time there. She had good memories of the place, but her partner, Henry, wasn't in favor of the business and she needed his approval. She invited me the following week to discuss it with him at their home.

They lived in a spacious apartment by the Seine with a stunning view of the Eiffel Tower. She and I sat around a small antique table in a corner of the living room while waiting for the others to join us. I had asked my accountant Alex to join us, but when Henry walked in, he wanted to get started straight away. He wore a crisp white shirt with the top button undone and trailed a sharp scent of citrus cologne. He took a seat, ran a hand through his wet hair, and focused his steady eyes on me. "I'm not in favor of this. There's no money in it."

I hadn't expected his immediate objection but came prepared. "I can show you the financials. Or my accountant can walk you—"

"I've already read them."

"We turned a profit a year ago—"

"Your three-year average was negative. Anyway, Silvia doesn't have time for a business, she needs to take care of our daughter."

He turned to her, and she cast her eyes down. He sat back and focused on me. "Look, we're not going to pay you a dime for this business. If Silvia insists on going ahead, we'll need you to stay around until the end of September."

I swallowed and looked at my watch. I needed Alex's help.

By the time he arrived, Henry had left. Alex pulled out a stack of documents from his satchel and spoke about the success of a small business surviving ten years. "All it needs is a bit more marketing."

Silvia's expression softened. Her professional background was PR. She wanted to know her dream had a chance.

On the bus ride home, I phoned Rachel to update her on the meeting. She was confident a deal was still possible; Henry hadn't said no.

That evening, I called Silvia to make a counteroffer. She could have the business for free, but we needed to sign an agreement by the end of July. The summer months were slow, and I would split the risk with her, but I couldn't stay longer; I needed to move on. Giving her a yoga studio that had been running for ten years at no cost was an enticing offer.

I heard noise in the background, and she said she would speak with Henry and get back to me.

"I can't stay tied to the past. Do you understand? It's because of Arun."

She called me the next day and said Henry had reluctantly agreed to go ahead.

ON THE LAST Monday of July, days from the planned sale of the business, the doorbell rang while I was getting ready for work. I wasn't expecting anyone, and the intercom hadn't buzzed. I padded to the front entrance in bare feet, looked through the peephole, and shrank back. Arun was standing behind the glass in his short-sleeved cotton shirt and jeans, the green duffel bag beside him. His familiar form eclipsed the eight months he had been away. What was he doing here? How did this happen? Could I get away without answering? No: he must have heard me come to the door and sensed my presence. I opened it a few inches.

The sweet dusty smell of his skin, concentrated from hours of travel, hit me with overwhelming recognition. With his hands in his pockets, he looked like an innocent child.

I seized control of my mind and shook off his presence like a warm blanket on a cold morning. "What are you doing here?"

His eyes settled on mine, as if he had been lost and just found home.

I clutched the doorknob. "I'm sorry but I can't let you in."

He waited for me to say something else, but no other words came.

"Let me use the bathroom at least."

I clung to the door for support. "Sorry."

It felt wrong to deny him a basic human need, but if I let him in, I couldn't be sure he would leave. He might stay against my will, overpower me physically. Regaining my space had been a hard-won battle, like pulling off a jellyfish. Suddenly my mind cleared. This was a trap; he was a trap.

"I'm sorry." I willed my arms to close the door, then walked to the bedroom on the other side of the apartment.

I called Trevor first, and he asked me to get in touch with Dad who offered to send his maid to stay with me as long as Arun was around.

Then I called Surat. He said Arun had left Rishikesh at dawn the day before without informing anyone, and reassured me he would help. "Don't worry. I call him. I take care."

Still on high alert, I waited a few minutes and took a few deep breaths. Then I picked up my work bag and tiptoed back to the entrance, shoes in hand. I looked through the peephole again: the landing was empty. I slipped on my shoes and took the elevator down in case Arun was in the staircase. His green bag lay unattended in the entrance hall. I picked it up and left it outside the building. Like closing the door in his face, it felt wrong, but he needed to know he wasn't welcome anywhere in my space.

As soon as I reached my office, I called Angela.

Her voice was charged, in a good way for once. "Why?"

"I don't know."

We assumed he would go to City Yoga, and she promised to tell me if he showed up there. I also called Silvia to warn her about Arun's unexpected appearance. I didn't want anything to upset the transfer of the business on Friday.

Surat called that afternoon. He had spoken with Arun: he would be back in India in a week. I hoped he was right.

For the next few days, I thought I might hear from Arun or he would show up at City Yoga, but strangely, he stayed away. His unplanned arrival on my doorstep was his only attempt to connect. It was a relief, of course. If he had realized the timing of his visit, he might have tried to interfere with the sale. But he seemed oddly indifferent to the place we had built together, the one I had worked so hard to keep for him. He didn't contact Angela, either. What had he traveled all the way to Paris for? Had he hoped to win me over in person? I could never be sure what he wanted from me, but the sooner I was free of City Yoga —and of him—the better.

On the morning of the sale, Silvia called and demanded a last-minute payment to cover unused classes. The company account was depleted, and I stood firm. When we met at her lawyer's office, her husband Henry was adamant that the payment was due, but I wasn't about to change our original agreement on the day of the sale. They were buying my business for nothing, and I was done with being pushed around. I made my position clear to Marc, who was also my lawyer for this transaction.

The lawyers suggested that Silvia and I have some time alone, and with the men out of the room, I convinced her to go ahead. The property agent arrived and joined us around the table. He gave Silvia a new lease to sign and pulled out the original document with my personal guarantee on the rent. He crossed out my signature and countersigned it, releasing me from the crushing financial obligation of the past ten years. He rolled his eyes at Silvia, but I didn't care; he was the instrument of my freedom, and I sent him a silent blessing.

When we all got up to leave, Henry shot me a look of disdain, but he might as well have kissed me. What had felt impossible was done. I flew all the way home.

36

MAIDEN NAME

Mid-September, six weeks after he showed up at my door, Arun sat with Surat in the waiting room of the municipal court. Dad was with Marc, a gap away from the others in the same row. I arrived with Aileen, Dad's maid, who had come to stay with me again during Arun's visit. I took a seat across from Arun, and she sat next to me. He and I acknowledged each other in silence. For the first time since Id' known him, he'd dyed his hair black, and though the sleek color lifted his appearance, it surprised me that a master of his physical longevity had resorted to such a common trick. On the day of our divorce, he looked good, but it was fake.

He stared at me, and his eyes misted. Aileen leaned in and whispered, "Let's sit somewhere else." We went to sit in a waiting room down the hall. "He was trying to hypnotize you. I could see it in his eyes."

Was that the game he played? Hypnotize me into caring for him? I prayed that it would all be over soon, and I was grateful that Surat was there. I had bought them both plane tickets and sent Surat an invitation to obtain a French visa, but within days of their trip, he still hadn't received it. As it seemed increasingly unlikely that he would be able to travel, he told me to be careful with Arun. He had been possessed by a spirit, become violent, and tried to hit Teju. Surat told me not to be alone with him. He had never uttered a word against Arun, and I took his counsel to heart. Then to my relief, his visa came through.

Aileen and I didn't have to wait long. Surat came to fetch us, and we trooped down a corridor and waited in front of the judge's office. She asked who wanted to go first, and I went in. She covered a few administrative questions, then asked if I was divorcing by mutual consent.

"Yes."

It was that simple.

When it was Arun's turn, I prayed he would understand the judge in French and give the same answer. He came out a couple of minutes later, and she handed Marc a thick document. Then she turned to our party with an open expression. "You're all done."

A few words had concluded months of effort. Eighteen years since I met Arun, our marriage had ended, and I was free from him.

We walked to the main entrance, and I welcomed the distraction of Surat posing in front of marble backdrops to have his photo taken in the French courthouse. Back on the street in the afternoon light, I was too stunned to think, but when Marc suggested a coffee across the street, I felt relieved. I needed a transition to close off my long relationship with Arun.

Dad and Mark sat at one table, while the rest of us shared the one behind them. Arun faced me with Surat beside him and Aileen next to me. I had no feelings against Arun. He was as familiar as an old friend, but I could now sit with him without worrying about what he might do or what he might ask for. I had earned this moment.

When our coffees arrived, he pushed the sugar toward me.

I slid it back. "I don't take sugar anymore."

He dropped a couple of cubes into his own cup and insisted, "It will taste better with sugar."

I shook my head. Already he no longer knew me.

After half an hour or so, Marc got up and said he was leaving with Dad, and we followed them out. Dad kissed me and walked away with Marc.

I turned to Arun. "We're taking the metro back. Do you want to come with us?"

"No, we'll take a cab."

As I watched Arun and Surat merge into the crowd, Aileen touched my arm. "He doesn't love you. He didn't turn to look back."

Of course not. Why would he? I had extracted myself from him. My account was closed, and he had to pursue his whims on his own.

As soon as I reached home, I turned on my phone and found a text message from Angela. "Is it over?"

I typed back. "Yes, thank God."

Her answer came right away. "Thank God, indeed."

Aileen and I ate leftovers for dinner; I took Arun's seat, the one that looked out toward the living room. It occurred to me that I should have planned a more celebratory meal, but I had been too preoccupied with the outcome of the day. I hadn't known until the last minute if everything would work out and Arun would go along with my plan. Alone in my bedroom that night, it was enough to be free.

The following morning, I asked Aileen to take a final bag of Arun's belongings to his hotel. On his arrival, she had delivered his suitcase of clothes, and he had called to ask if there was anything else; he was sure he had left more behind. She had returned with cheap gifts from him: a garland of fake marigolds and a common essential oil. I had asked him for only one item from Rishikesh: a bottle of rose oil I had bought there years ago and hadn't found anywhere elsewhere. It wasn't very expensive

—nothing compared to all the money and goods he had from me over the years—but he had brought a cheap alternative. And what was he thinking with the plastic flowers? It would have been better if he had brought nothing.

In this last bag I had packed his etched silver opium holders and a 3D stereoscopic photo viewer, antiques he had all the way back from when I first met him in Rishikesh. He had been so excited to show me the viewer—how flat slides turned into 3D images—but despite several attempts, I still couldn't see what he saw. These objects had survived our moves to Fontainebleau, Paris, Valbonne, Maidenhead, and our return to Paris. It had crossed my mind to keep them—small prizes for all he had taken—but then I decided I didn't want anything of his.

I also asked Aileen to take Lily and Benny along for a final goodbye. As we were making divorce plans, Arun had asked for Benny, but I told him they came as a pair. When I quoted the cost of sending them to India, he said I could keep them. I was grateful they were still with me.

As soon as the door shut behind Aileen, I felt a sudden urge to go with her. I swallowed and sat at my desk. What was I thinking? We were divorced now and had already said our final goodbyes. I breathed through the knot in my belly.

When she returned, I asked her how it went.

"Fine. He didn't say anything. Took the bag."

"Did he pet Lily and Benny?"

"Only Benny. He took him in his arms and held him."

His dog. "You know, I was tempted to go with you. Bring the dogs myself to say goodbye."

She paused. "I know. You still love him. It's the same with my ex-husband. He hurt me, but I still look at his photos on Facebook."

No: it wasn't love. It was the pain of tearing down my past.

I needed time to process the change, but the real break had taken place earlier in the spring when I changed my surname back to Tamraz. Years before I had gladly accepted Arun's name as mine and relinquished my father's name and its associations. But now, at the age of forty, I took possession of my maiden name anew. It wasn't exclusively Dad's; it wasn't even obviously Lebanese. It belonged to my ancestors and was a link to the people and places I had been born into. No matter how much I had wanted to reject my past, I wasn't Indian, and I wasn't a yogi.

ONCE I WAS free of Arun, I needed to have one more conversation. I didn't look forward to it but had to do it: it was another reparation. The naked ceiling bulb lit the green walls of the dining room, and my heart pounded in my chest. I hadn't heard from Angela since the day of the divorce a couple of weeks earlier. The room was quiet, and I forced myself to breathe while I pressed the button and waited.

Her voice sounded wary when she answered.

"It's me."

"I know. I wasn't expecting you to call."

"How are you?"

"As good as can be expected. Under the circumstances."

I didn't know what she meant, but she was in *that* sort of mood. Silence weighed the line, and I shifted in my seat. "I wanted to apologize."

"For what? You don't need to apologize to me."

"Yes. I do. I should have protected you. From him." My voice was raw at first, then grew stronger as I spoke. "I should have never let those things happen."

"You didn't need to protect me. I knew what I was doing." She sounded wise now, but she had been scared then.

"I should have. I'm sorry."

"I've already gone through it in therapy. I know why it happened."

What had she discussed in therapy? Had she uncovered the reasons for becoming involved with a married couple? She didn't say more, and I didn't want to pry.

"I should have done more to stop it," I said.

She was quiet for a moment, then her voice came out soft, almost intimate. "I knew those spirits."

She spoke as if she were revealing an important personal secret, but what did she mean by "know"? Tao, Udo—they had entered my life with Arun and left with him. They belonged to him and to his world, and I couldn't claim to know them.

Her admission caught me off-guard, and I was still pondering it when she took on a breezy tone. "It's all over now. Let's not think about it anymore." She had let her guard down, said more than she intended, and didn't want me to linger there.

"I'm planning to get a new email." She paused. "I don't know if you want to stay in touch. I'll send you a message when I have it."

I sensed she wouldn't.

When we hung up, our conversation left me as unsatisfied as so many others before. What had I expected from her? Tears? An epiphany? An apology of her own?

Later, when the immediate effect had passed, what remained with me was the deathly timbre of her voice when she evoked the spirits. As if they were a challenge to life itself.

SHORTLY AFTER THEIR return to Rishikesh, Surat called to say Arun was planning to sell our house. I reminded him that half the property belonged to me.

"House is not in your name. Very difficult."

"What about the divorce settlement?"

"Not official property. Use only. Not possible for you. Foreigner."

I digested his words. The land was held through "squatters' rights," I knew that, but I hadn't appreciated that the property was excluded from me as a foreigner. Arun had bought it in his name and bequeathed it to me in his will, but Surat implied the document was useless. I had shared everything with Arun and assumed he had safeguarded my interests in the same way, but I had clearly been misguided.

To be sure I had understood, I asked Surat, "So, he'll get all the money from any sale?"

"Yes. Don't worry. I buy it."

"You want the house?"

"I buy it and pay him your money."

"Forty thousand euros?"

"Yes. Leftover I keep for you."

Surat was offering me a way to extract my share of the property and pay my divorce settlement to Arun. Although I had been able to save money since he left, there had been another set of unexpected taxes after the divorce. Surat's offer made sense.

Arun had already been in touch several times asking for his money, but I was in no rush to speak with him. The next time he called I confronted him about selling the house behind my back and brought up Surat's offer.

"Surat's trying to cheat us. He's offering a very low price. I can get more. As soon as I sell it, I promise I'll send you your share."

"No, you won't. My name's not on the property documents."

"When are you sending my money?"

"I told you, Surat will pay you from my share of the house."

"Jo, I miss you. Why are you punishing me like this?" He broke down into loud sobs.

I couldn't believe he was at it again and mimicked his sounds. "You think you're the only one who can cry?"

He stopped cold. Not even a murmur disturbed the line. When we hung up, I stared at the silent object on the dining table. All this time he had been acting.

He called again a couple of days later and put on his mopey voice again as if he had never been caught out. Each word twisted my belly. "I have a buyer for the house."

"What about Surat?"

'He's offering me much less."

"I already told you, Surat will buy it and pay my settlement to you."

"But you're still sending me the money?"

"Arun, how many times do I need to say the same thing? I am not sending money. Surat will give it to you from my share of the house."

"You promised to send me the cash after the divorce."

"But half of the house is mine."

"I promise you, Jo, I have a good buyer. He's offering ten million rupees."

Close to our investment of two hundred thousand euros. Surat's offer was twenty percent lower, but he would let Arun live there for the rest of his life. And I couldn't tell if Arun was telling the truth. He might not have a buyer at all.

He put on a mellifluous tone. "Believe me, Jo, I won't cheat you." After a pause, he added, "We used to be friends, right?"

Friends: the word, startlingly pure, threw me back to our early days together. Was that how he saw me now? He had been my teacher, lover, husband—we were supposed to be soul mates, bound to each other across lifetimes. Friends didn't come close to describing what we had been to each other. The term was wrong, and it hurt. Yet he sounded tender and measured, and I wanted to believe him and sell the house at the best price.

Then I regained control of my mind: this man was a shapeshifter; I couldn't let myself be swayed by him. It tore me to say it, but I stood firm. "Sorry Arun. I'm going with Surat."

It was our last conversation.

Surat sent me written confirmation that I had fulfilled the terms of our divorce agreement, and I never heard from Arun again.

37

LIFTING THE VEIL

A few weeks later, on a November evening when the air was newly cold, Trevor called me on his drive home from work as he did most days, and asked if I had heard from Arun. Night had fallen early, and the apartment was still.

"No, nothing. Once he realized there was no more money coming from me, he stopped calling."

"Good."

His response was sensible, but a question nagged at my mind. Arun had flipped so suddenly from incessant calling to complete silence, and I let it slip without forethought.

"Do you think he ever loved me?"

As soon as the words left my mouth, they sounded absurd; and I knew—as clear as one picture replacing another. Images flashed across my mind. Arun opening the door, bewildered and weary, for my first yoga class at dawn. Tao standing by the crate of wine in the mountain house, a grin on his face. Arun tottering in the darkened kitchen in Fontainebleau, eyeing me with suspicion, preparing for a showdown. The sheen of his black hair at the courthouse, eyes misted over. Every moment of our life had been a sham. He never had any intention of giving me half the house in India; he had used me every step of the way. He had been a mastermind, and I had been his fool. All at once—irrevocably—his mask fell.

"Oh my God, he never loved me."

Trevor's breathing on the line drew me back to the present.

"I'm sorry," he said. "I didn't know how to tell you. I didn't know when we would ever talk about it."

Sobs of shame, anger, regret engulfed me. "So what did he want? What did he ever want from me?"

"You're going to be fine, love. You're stronger than this. It's called lifting the veil."

The following morning, I wrote a formal letter to the French Department of Immigration about our divorce and requested the cancellation of Arun's residency card.

When I returned to New York for Christmas, I met Letty, our childhood nanny, for lunch. After she retired from working for our family she and I stayed close, and I visited her each time I went home. I asked her about her life before she moved to the US, and although she didn't pry, she knew about my problematic marriage to Arun. This time, I told her about the divorce and my new relationship with Trevor.

I could see she was happy, but she didn't say much until I walked her back to her building. As I was about to leave, she gripped my arm with her gnarled arthritic hand and drew me in, close enough for me to smell her powdery lilac perfume. Her voice dropped to a whisper. "I've been praying for you every day." Her piercing eyes met mine. "That you would meet a good man. One who will love you and take care of you."

As she brushed the tears from her cheek, I swallowed the lump in my throat and thanked her for her prayers.

Surat called with the news that Arun had given most of the cash from the sale of the house to his son. He sounded concerned, and although I was grateful for his confidence and continued friendship, Arun's choices had nothing to do with me. He could dispose of his money as he saw fit.

I didn't hear from Surat again until a few months later when he told me that Arun had booked a flight to Paris but was denied a visa at the French Consulate in Delhi. I was relieved to hear that my letter had been effective and he wouldn't be able to come back and hurt other women. I breathed easier after that.

A YEAR and a half after my divorce, I joined Trevor in the UK.

A COUPLE of months after my move, I received a final message from Arun through Facebook. He had lost his ability to spell and asked me why I had abandoned him after he left his "fem-lay" for me.

EARLY ON IN my relationship with Arun, Dad had said to me, "Why did he choose you? What did you have? Fifty thousand maybe? He could have gone for someone with millions." At the time his logic shocked me; his easy dismissal of the man I loved and who loved me back.

But his assessment was off the mark. He didn't consider what it would have been like to grow up poor in India in the fifties. If Arun's origin story held a kernel of truth and he had indeed lost his parents during partition, being an orphan would have been a further disadvantage. Fifty thousand dollars would have been a significant sum—as indeed it would be for most people—and that was only the beginning.

As I look back at photos of Arun, it strikes me that he was always posing. Staring daringly at the camera; parting his lips in the hint of a smile; elegant and sleek; convinced of his irresistibility. He may not have succeeded as an actor in India, but he deployed his talents in Los Angeles. Marrying the words of love with the thrall of enlightenment, he perfected the tools of his trade: seduction, deception, and manipulation. He found the perfect prey—sensitive women he could woo passionately and swindle gently—while convincing them that they were loved by a good man.

When he moved from LA to northern California at the age of fifty-one, his lucky streak came to an abrupt end. Or perhaps his golden period had always been paid for with borrowed time, his debt to the spirits mounting. When the teenage girls told their story, they accused him of the game he had played for years: abuse of the unassuming.

In prison, he obtained his high school equivalency degree and discovered novels, beyond his usual fare of newspapers. He read and spoke. But on his release, he lost not only his livelihood but his green card. Back in India, even his old wife didn't want him.

It was an Englishman who first took him to Rishikesh, and in the holy town of the yogis, where incense perfumes the air and dreams take the shape of reality, he donned the orange color of the swamis. Who would question his past?

One afternoon, when he had been there a year, as he sat by the Ganges at twilight, a young woman, barely older than a girl, appeared. In her devotion he saw his opportunity; mirroring her beliefs and promising her unconditional love—the fulfillment of her deepest need. Even he didn't envision how far she would go to turn his luck.

Growing up I didn't know Dad. He was nothing like my best friend's father, or the cultural ideal of the protective parent. He inhabited my life in brief moments stolen from everyday routine. I couldn't make sense of how he operated, and this absence of understanding left me with anxious questions. Mom loved and hated him at the same time. She was shocked when he had children with another partner during their marriage, but that's not why she finally left him.

When I first met Arun, he seemed like the opposite of Dad: strong, dark, present; dangerous to men, loving to women. We were two sides of the same coin, and he would never leave me. I wanted so much to believe I had found the one; even when it was clear that he wasn't, I couldn't give up my ideal. After I left him, Mom told me that while I was with him she had feared for my life, but reasoned that he depended on me and wouldn't destroy his source.

I paid a high price for my idealism, and I was lucky to escape. It could have been much worse. For years, he plundered money—several hundred thousand dollars—for his investments in India and bought jewelry for himself, not to mention what he took from me. But finance is only the most rudimentary form of accounting. For years, he absorbed my energy while I remained in his thrall, distanced from family and friends who wondered what had happened to the woman they once knew. I would have given up anything for Tao and Arun to give up their double life, for Arun to be exclusively mine again—but now I am grateful every day that his mask fell. The tragedy wasn't that he got me but that I was lost to myself for so long.

I was twenty-two when I met him—eager for all the world had to offer, but also apprehensive about my role in it. His promise of deeper secret knowledge was alluring; his allusion to the spiritual masters he served intriguing. By the time we moved to the UK when I was twenty-six, I struggled to find my footing amid his changing moods and schemes. A decade later, on the verge of losing my job, as I took stock of everything I had accomplished, I became aware of my own power. With Arun there was no firm base to stand on, and had I stayed I would have continued to balance on the edge of a precipice.

I was an easy target. My beliefs in Baba, the elders, Tao, and the potential of enlightenment formed the mental chains with which he held me. Past lives, reincarnation, and soul mates were its links. Now these words sound like empty instruments of control.

The word yoga comes from the same root as the word yoke —to tie together. It first occurs in the *Rig Veda,* the most ancient Hindu scripture (c. 1500-1200 BCE) where it usually refers to the yoking of two animals. This link can be a positive form of connection, but it can also be a dangerous bondage. The very fluidity around yoga's meaning invites manipulation, starting with the origin myth that yoga is a sacred practice created in India millennia ago. This statement is repeated de facto when yoga is mentioned, despite Mark Singleton's detailed demonstration in *Yoga Body* that the exercises practiced today do not come from ancient texts, but rather were developed at the turn of the twentieth century from foreign and local elements. Whatever the claims may be, the physical practice has no inherent spiritual merit. The master chooses the rules.

Arun is far from unique among the yoga gurus of our time. Take Bikram Choudhury, his old pal and creator of a trademarked hot yoga sequence. He built a global empire around his person and brand, accumulating significant wealth, while behind the scenes he led a different life and was accused of sexual abuse by multiple women. He fled from the US, where he faces criminal charges. Yoga did not make him good.

Bikram is not alone. Gurus of the other major branches of yoga have also been accused of sexual abuse, most notably Pattabhi Jois, founder of the hugely influential Ashtanga yoga, from which all subsequent flow-based yogas were created. Similar allegations have been made against senior swamis of Sivananda Ashram and Yogi Bhajan, originator of the widespread Kundalini yoga. Arun knew of all these men, and imagined perhaps that he could float above them.

Not all forms of abuse are graphic. While I was still living in

Paris, Vanessa and I attended a workshop on "yoga nidra" (yoga of sleep) as a special treat for her birthday. We left the class intrigued by our experience of lucid sleep, but by the time I reached home I felt out of sorts, and the sensation of being off lingered until the next morning. I spoke with Vanessa about it, and she reported having lain on the couch in a grouchy mood for the rest of the evening after the workshop. When I told Mom about being induced into a lucid sleep, she recognized it as hypnosis and expressed disapproval at the instructor's lack of transparency and integrity. I had no idea what I was venturing into upon signing up for the workshop. How many other people fall into the practice unaware of being hypnotized?

Even after my divorce, out of habit or enjoyment, I continued to start the day as I had for years, sitting cross-legged on the Tibetan rug. I dropped my chin to my chest and focused on my breathing—the controlled inhale, the pause, then the drawn-out exhale—harnessing my thoughts to my breath. But as weeks turned to months, and my life evolved in a different direction, the habit loosened. I started to skip days until finally I stopped altogether. It simply did not make sense anymore. Why was I still practicing what Arun had taught me under false pretenses?

The secret practice wasn't secret. The principles of Agni Yoga, the yoga of fire, come from Chinese meditation styles and can also be found in cryptic medieval Hatha Yoga texts. Contracting the pelvic muscles is also known as Kegel exercises. Similarly, the TM mantras, my first introduction to meditation, are also falsely presented as bespoke when in fact they're set by age group. Their power is supposed to derive from their secrecy, but this is a tool to control the devotee. Arun spoke of his martial arts training, preferred judo mats for physical practice, and carried some of the strength of his past, but I never saw him practicing meditation.

Yogis in ancient India were bands of men who lived outside the caste system. They spent time in cemeteries, covered themselves in funeral ash, and flouted religious injunctions against eating meat, drinking wine, and having sex outside marriage. Feared as immoral black magicians, they remind me of Arun.

Before meeting him, I didn't believe in evil. I had studied the state-led horrors of twentieth-century Europe both at school and at university, but these historical events seemed far from my own experience. Living with him I witnessed firsthand his insatiable desires, deep restlessness, and haunting emptiness. As if nothing in life would ever matter. While I no longer believe in a spirit called Tao who had once been my brother and Arun's best friend, I know Arun harbored and spawned destructive forces.

While meditation can indeed calm the mind, extraordinary claims about long life, choosing one's time of death, and obtaining otherworldly insight are illusions created to ensnare —deceptive claims that are also at the heart of Transcendental Meditation and its promotion of mindless yogic hopping. When the time came to leave Arun, the answers didn't come to me from meditation; the practice didn't show me the way out.

Arun was a waste of time; the yoga school was not. To his mirage, I joined my drive and passion to help others. He forbade the teaching of spiritual elements (such as reciting a mantra or a Sanskrit prayer), and our teaching team was sincere. They cared for the clients' well-being, many of whom will retain the positive spirit with which we taught physical and breathing exercises.

When I regained my own space, I yearned to explore the world outside the confines of the yoga mat. I went to Zumba classes and cycled in the Bois de Boulogne. I rediscovered the wonders of movement, three-dimensional space, nature.

My years in the colorful world of yoga have made me wary of calm flowing voices and flowery language promising to soothe my mind and heal my body. Now when I feel like stretching, I simply stretch. To build strength, I focus on movements and do the work. I don't want or need an additional spiritual narrative to distract me from my own experience. I paid a high price for my faith, and I was fortunate to escape with my mind intact, though traumatized. It took me years to find freedom: I won't give away my power again.

I don't regret obtaining my MBA, my years in the corporate world, and of course, meeting Trevor. The path of my youth forged me, but I am grateful every day I am no longer on it. Emptying my mind is not my goal. A blank mind isn't a cure. Closing my eyes doesn't make me good. Meditation doesn't replace morality.

I have returned to my Judeo-Christian roots to guide me in what is essentially and irrevocably a moral world. The quiet I once sought in meditation I now find in prayer. For my wrongs, I seek forgiveness and practice repentance. The universe is alive and teeming with possibilities, and if I don't exercise my moral obligation through action, someone else will do it for me.

38

TWO YEARS LATER

I miss Surat's call, but I already know what he will say. I haven't heard from Arun since his Facebook message, and he has left my conscious mind. He only appears from time to time in my dreams, hovers over me like a wraith, and smothers my life energy. The fear I never felt for him in life surges at night. Sometimes it's not even his face I see, but a dark form, and I awake to a primal scream.

Surat doesn't wait for me to return his call and sends a text: "Arun-ji dead."

I phone him immediately. "When?"

"Last night."

"What happened?"

"Infection."

"Was he sick?"

"Yes. Bad infection."

I want to know more: How long was he sick? Did he suffer? What did he say in his final moments? But there is only so much Surat can tell me in English, so I ask, "Were you still friends? At the end?"

"Yes, yes. Always friends."

There is nothing more to say, and we end the conversation. I step out of my home office and walk into the bedroom. As my eyes scan the view of the hills in the distance, my mind drifts and I am in Rishikesh.

Arun is lying on the mahogany bed in the vast master bedroom. His eyes are closed. Fine white hair frames his face. His thin aquiline nose is still. Not a single breath; no flicker of life animates his body. The thick mattress engulfs him. He is reduced by death.

My twenty-two-year-old self appears by his side. The yellow muslin tunic she took so much pleasure in choosing catches the light. She has been gone so long, it's good to see her. In the prime of life, she has decided that she will love this man forever. Nothing in the world—neither her mother's warnings nor her father's wrath—will separate them. She is so sure of herself her smile cannot be extinguished.

I take this girl's shoulders, pull her away from him, and hold her in my arms. Tears wet my face. She is naïve—yet so innocent. She has no right to smile. No right to love this way. Believe an older man's lies. Succumb to his ruse.

But today he is gone. The man who claimed to know the way to physical longevity and taught her to repeat, "I will not die, I will leave my body," died at the age of seventy-six. And she is alive.

I let him go and forgive him. Once again. Completely. Forgive myself.

ACKNOWLEDGMENTS

They say it takes a village to create something as complex as a book; it also takes a series of felicitous encounters.

I discovered the power of journaling and developed a passion for life writing in my eighth-grade English class with Christine Schutt. I owe her a debt of gratitude for paying attention to my words and setting me on the writing path.

Since the time of my divorce, I knew I wanted to write this story, but it would take me five years to find a way into it. I'm grateful to Sally Davies for encouraging me to write out of sheer enjoyment when I doubted my own ability.

A latch opened in my mind and memories began to spill out at a writing day in Chris Leonard's summer garden. Chris saw potential in my work, and I'm thankful that she invited me to join her Write On critique group at a time when I needed discipline and structure.

My memoir was significantly transformed by the insights of my beta readers. I'd like to thank Jill Witty, who provided generous and perceptive observations, notably on the importance of the parental roles; Heather Lanfermeijer, who pointed out gaps in the narrative; and Rosie Passi, a friend during and beyond the Arun years, who gave me early feedback and encouraged me to tell a difficult story.

Long ago, I was lucky enough to share an elementary school classroom with Melissa Mueller. Muse extraordinaire, she sparked my youthful curiosity and ignited my love of words. Our decades-long friendship brings me joy, and I'm grateful for her discerning beta reading and lightning-quick editing of my first query package.

My book has benefited greatly from the work of exceptional professionals. Amber Hatch provided valuable feedback on my writing style and story structure. Thanks to her I remember to favor punchy sentences.

Richard Arcus steered my book in the right direction and reflected the essence of my story in his sensitive and astute observations, edits, and back cover copy. Working with him gave me the confidence to publish independently. I'm grateful for his professional approach and encouragement.

Jennifer Duardo completed a meticulous and thorough proofread and provided significant copy edits. Her sharp eye and efficient process made the final editing of my book a smooth and seamless experience.

I was very fortunate to work with Kari Brownlie on my cover design. She was patient and responsive throughout the process and created a beautiful cover.

My writing journey would have been much lonelier and far less fruitful without my online writing community: the #writingcommunity and #5amwritersclub on Twitter—a full force of inspiration and encouragement. Special thanks to Ralph Walker for bringing us together on video meetups, helping us to develop into a closer group of supportive writers.

The band of Subversive Feminist Mermaids—Amy, Ellen, Ev, Gail, Jess, and Nancy—lift me up with their presence, friendship, and writerly wisdom. Dana Goldstein reached out to me and offered her advice early on. Karen DeBonis shared her marketing toolkit and enthusiasm. Maria Daversa lit the path of independent publishing and extended a helping hand with more kindness than I could have hoped for. Jean Brown connected with the purpose of my story, offered her support, and wrote a validating editorial review. My UK Writing and Marketing group brought camaraderie on the journey, and my conversations with Lucy Weldon over tea and cake brightened key junctures and inspired the opening paragraph of my book. I could not have hoped for better friends and colleagues in my second career.

Outside the writing world, I am indebted to Rachel and Vanessa. Their kindness and support carried me through a life-changing time. I will never forget the role they played in my recovery.

I'm blessed every day by the love of my family. Mom—not only my mother but also my close friend and fellow memoir writer: the journey wouldn't have been half as enjoyable without you. Dad—you were there when I needed you, whether I recognized it or not at the time; you passed on your love of books and expressed genuine excitement when I told you about my memoir. My siblings—Sabrina, answer to my first deep wish, Eduardo, and Margherita: I'm lucky to have you in my life.

Trevor—my life partner and fellow adventurer: I am deeply grateful for your unwavering conviction, enthusiasm, and support at each step of the way. Thank you for believing in me and my story before I did.

ABOUT THE AUTHOR

Joelle Tamraz has been putting pen to paper ever since she learned about journaling in her eighth-grade English class. She worked in large technology companies as a business manager and director for two decades and owned a yoga studio for ten years. She holds an Honors BA in social studies from Harvard and an MBA from INSEAD. She is also a certified life coach and a youth mentor. She's passionate about sustainability and loves spending time outdoors, walking, cycling, or simply being in nature. *The Secret Practice* is her debut memoir.

For more information and additional resources, please visit her website: joelletamraz.com. If you'd like to be the first to receive her writing updates and subscriber specials, sign up for her newsletter: joelletamraz.com/newsletter-and-blog.

.

REVIEWS

If you enjoyed this book, please take a moment to post a review on Amazon and Goodreads. Reviews are so helpful for independent authors to have their books discovered by other readers. Thank you!

amazon.com

goodreads.com